W9-AWO-400

Prostate Cancer

SYLVAN MEYER
and
SEYMOUR C. NASH, M.D., F.A.C.S.

Prostate Cancer

Making Survival Decisions

THE UNIVERSITY OF CHICAGO PRESS

Chicago and London

SYLVAN MEYER has served as editor for the *Gainesville* (Georgia) *Times* and the *Miami News,* and was both editor and publisher of *South Florida Magazine,* which he founded in 1975. SEYMOUR C. NASH, M.D., is a fellow of the American College of Surgeons and a diplomate of the American Board of Urology. He is chairman of the Urology Department at Mt. Sinai Hospital, Miami Beach.

The University of Chicago Press, Chicago 60637
The University of Chicago Press, Ltd., London
© 1994 by The University of Chicago
All rights reserved. Published 1994
Printed in the United States of America
03 02 01 00 99 98 97 96 95 94   1 2 3 4 5
ISBN: 0-226-56857-1   (cloth)

LIBRARY OF CONGRESS CATALOGING-IN-PUBLICATION DATA

Meyer, Sylvan.
    Prostate cancer : making survival decisions / Sylvan Meyer and
Seymour C. Nash.
        p.   cm.
    Includes bibliographical references and index.
    1. Prostate—Cancer—Popular works.   I. Nash, Seymour C.
II. Title.
RC280.P7M49   1994
616.99'463—dc20   94-25487
                                                                CIP

♾ The paper used in this publication meets the
minimum requirements of the American National Standard
for Information Sciences—Permanence of Paper for
Printed Library Materials, ANSI Z39.48-1984.

With love and admiration
for their patience and support,
and for listening to endless conversations
about prostate cancer,
we dedicate this work to our wives,
ANNE MEYER and SALLY NASH

Contents

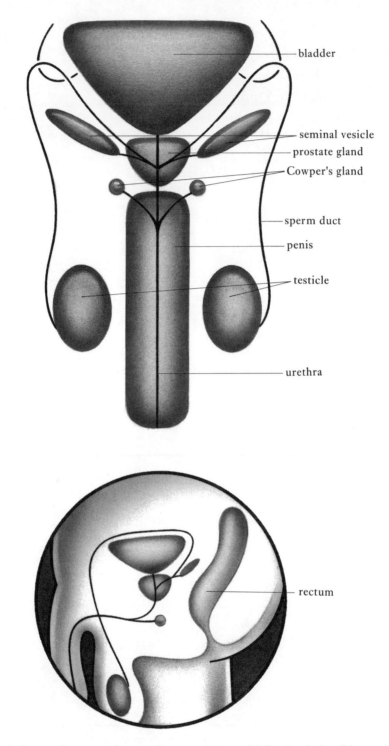

Schematic diagram of prostate and surrounding organs (not to scale). Drawings by Joan Swann.

Memo from Sylvan Meyer

When I found out I had prostate cancer, I wanted to learn everything about
   it I could.
What were they going to do to me and why?
What were the assorted treatments like? Would they hurt? Were they dan-
   gerous?
Would they leave me impaired? Would they leave me impotent?
What kind of research is going on? Have they discovered any new medicine
   or procedure that might increase my chances?
Would it kill me? If so, how long would it take?

I read several books about prostate cancer. They were about either one
man's excruciating personal and emotional experiences, or they were so
shallow they barely told me more than I had picked up from newspapers
and television. Or else they were written by doctors who talked so far down
to me I knew there was more to it than they were telling.

I wanted to know what the doctors know—the good, the bad—the in-
siders' ungarbled scoop. I wanted their inside info, how they looked on
their treatments and their patients; I even wanted their insider jokes.

Dr. Seymour (Cy) Nash, when he saw I was serious and could take the
information, good, bad, or indifferent, promised to help me and collabo-
rated on this book.

I have been studying prostate cancer off and on for almost four years.
I've been a newspaper and magazine editor and publisher for more than
forty years and a reporter all my life. I can't write about a complicated subject until I am sure I understand it and won't make any errors of fact or
interpretation. That's why it took so long. I am not saying the book isn't
controversial or that all the scientists involved in prostate cancer treatment
and research will agree with Cy and me. I do say, as a prostate cancer victim, there's a lot in here I wish I had known before I started treatment and
am glad I know after it.

Introduction

How I Got into All This

My Personal Experience

This book traces my personal experience with prostate cancer. I underwent thirty-eight days of radiation treatments. As with most radiation-treated patients I don't know for sure whether I am "cured," whether the cancer is permanently suppressed. I will be checked regularly.

Most books that I could find by laymen on this subject were highly emotional accounts of victims' personal ordeals, written at a time of little general knowledge of prostate cancer or of today's advanced treatment methods. However, I did not want to view my own cancer emotionally. I expected to beat it and would never put my family through the long, drawn-out ordeals described by these earlier fellow victims.

The purpose of this book is twofold: to inform the so-far unafflicted and undiagnosed about a disease that strikes 8 to 10 percent of adult American men and that concerns us all; and to help the diagnosed patient understand his problem and his options.

I hoped to write this book with a minimum of sentimentality, to pass along in lay terms what you need to know about the invader in your plumbing. To do that, the book explores prostate cancer from both the patient's and the physician's point of view. It covers some benign ailments of the prostate (but mostly is about cancer) and the details of what the surgeon thinks and sees as he performs various prostate surgeries. It reports on current treatment practices such as surgery, radiation, implanted seeds, cryosurgery, hormonal manipulations, and chemicals, and on various combinations of treatment strategies. You need to know what's happening to you and "what it is like" to go through the treatments.

I found a paucity of literature useful to patients and probable patients when I set out to write this book. Most is either out of date, too elementary, journalistically overcondensed or written by doctors for doctors. This is a serious work, the result of almost four years of research and study. However, I've tried not to make it heavy going, but readable, so that you can plunge without drowning into a medical subject that could affect your survival.

The book tracks my own experience, but no one patient would undergo every possible treatment and recovery routine, so Dr. Nash and I have relied on his observations as a physician and on the written and oral experiences of others. We have tried to organize the information so that you build understanding as you move along and develop enough background to ask intelligent and pertinent questions of your doctors and specialists. Our intention is to inform you objectively, not to disturb you needlessly nor to induce a false sense of security.

It's immediately apparent that your family will be deeply involved. The word cancer frightens them. Your wife or lady friend imagines the worst despite her attempts to cheer you and minimize the threat. You don't feel any different than you did the day before the news struck, but your children, probably grown up and with children of their own if you are of the average age of cancer discovery, show both concern and lack of knowledge about the disease. I assume you can take the bad news with the encouraging news, and there's more of the latter than you might think. You'll have to decide what to share with your family. You will find conflicting information and medical controversies concerning prostate cancer. If you, or your family, don't know the whole picture, fragments of information can be confusing —and troubling.

Learning on the grapevine I was writing about prostate cancer, a number of friends from around the country called to ask questions. They thought their questions too elementary or too stupid to put to their doctors. They were wrong: there are no stupid questions when your life is on the line. Their questions did tell me of the instant concerns of new prostate cancer patients.

Part 1 of this book deals primarily with my own experience and what you might expect in direct analysis and treatment. Part 2 is reportorial and technical rather than personal. Some chapters are extensions of information in part 1. It deals more deeply with information about prostate cancer and what science is doing about it. You don't necessarily have to read them in sequence; you might want to read portions of part 2 related to certain portions of part 1 before completing either part. Both parts serve our mission.

Our overarching purpose is to get you through prostate cancer treatment with knowledge and we hope success, or if you aren't a patient to get you to your urologist on a regular basis so if you are ever diagnosed you will catch your cancer while it can be tamed.

Don't panic. There are defenses against this cancer. There are huge ranges of differences in what it might do to particular men. You are in for some inconvenience and discomfort, but unless you are already in pain you have time to adjust to your new bodily companion and to keep control of your life. There are support groups of other victims who can reassure you. There's some helpful reading available to you from the American Cancer Society and other sources.

Your own attitude is important; let it rouse your fighting spirit and don't let it ruin your sense of humor. I agree with the late Norman Cousins (who did not die of prostate cancer) that a strong mental attitude and continued joy in life are damn good medicine for anything.

*   *   *

ONE MORE NOTE: This is a book of information, not direct nor specific medical advice. Only your doctor, knowing your individual circumstances, can advise you.

Acknowledgments

UNLESS WE INVADE a medical field on an obsessive mission, such as this one, lay people remain unaware of the huge and ongoing information exchanges among physicians and scientists. Dr. Nash and I deeply appreciate those professionals in teaching hospitals and in personal practices who devote untold time to research, to tracking assorted therapies and reporting their findings and to writing for the several general and special publications we have consulted in preparing this book. Such zeal could arise only from a sincere dedication to expanding knowledge in their professions.

In addition to their writings, several busy professionals generously gave us their time in both written and spoken exchanges. Our heartfelt thanks to Drs. Gary Ayers and Robert Tyrrel, Northside Hospital, Atlanta, Ga.; John C. Blasko, Northwest Tumor Institute, Seattle, Wa.; Charles B. Brendler, University of Chicago; Stanley Brosman, Santa Monica Urological Group, Santa Monica, Calif.; William Catalona, Washington University, St. Louis, Mo.; Jeffrey Cohen and Ralph Miller, Allegheny General Hospital, Pittsburgh, Pa.; William H. Cooner, Emory University, Atlanta, Ga.; Jean B. deKernion, UCLA School of Medicine, Los Angeles, Calif.; William A. Fair, Memorial Sloan-Kettering Cancer Center, New York, N.Y.; P. James Furlong, Miami Beach, Fla.; J. Arthur Heise (Ph.D.), dean of the School of Journalism and Mass Communication, Florida International University, Miami, Fla.; Fernand Labrie, Central Hospital of Laval University, Quebec, Canada; Timothy McHugh, St. Joseph Mercy Hospital, Ann Arbor, Mich.; James L. Montie, Wayne State University Medical School, Detroit, Mich.; Gerald L. Murphy, Tumor Institute, Seattle, Wash.; David Paulson, Duke University Medical School, Durham, N.C.; Donald G. Skinner, University of Southern California Medical Center, Los Angeles, Calif.; Thomas A. Stamey, Stanford University Medical Center, Stanford, Calif.; Leonard Toonkel, Mt. Sinai Medical Center, Miami Beach, Fla.; Andrew von Eschenbach, University of Texas M. D. Anderson Medical Center, Houston, Tx.; Patrick C. Walsh, Johns Hopkins University, Baltimore, Md.; Willet F. Whitmore Jr.,

Memorial Sloan-Kettering Cancer Center, New York, N.Y.; Horst
Zincke, Mayo Clinic, Rochester, Mn.

Special thanks to the following: Marvin Silverstein, M.D., Atlanta, retired chief of Radiology at Northside Hospital, lifelong friend, and personal medical advisor, constructive critic of medical writing efforts, and
constant guide and interpreter through medical vocabularies and pro-
clivities; Ed Estes, M.D., and Frank G. Lake III, M.D., urologist and radiologist respectively of Northeast Georgia Regional Medical Center,
Gainesville, Ga., for helpful read-through and specific advice; Leslie R.
Schover, Ph.D., Cleveland Clinic Foundation, Cleveland, Ohio, for specific counsel and copy-correcting of the potency chapter; Ivy Edwards,
University of Miami Journalism Department and now returned to New-
port Beach, New South Wales, Australia, for vital assistance in research
and medical library sleuthing; Congresswoman Ileana Ros-Lehtinen (R-
Fla.) for general encouragement; and David Lang, Atlanta, Ga., for raising
the tough questions.

Grateful acknowledgment of help on the part of University of Miami
and Mt. Sinai Medical Center libraries, and from various doctors' staff
members for arrangements and patience, especially the staff of Dr. Nash,
Barbara Pratt and Flora Gonzales, who were involved in "literary" as well
as medical services to co-author Meyer; also to staff and officials of the
American Cancer Society, the National Institutes of Health, the National
Cancer Institute, and other organizations; to the several unnamed fellow
victims of prostate cancer who shared their experiences with us.

This book would have been impossible without the meticulous copy-
reading of Louis R. Fockele, Gainesville, Ga., former publisher of the
Gainesville, Ga., *Times*, and valued longtime friend and associate; or the
focused editorial counsel of former University of North Carolina school-
mate Ernest Frankel, Los Angeles, Calif. (you got it, Lou—a fraternity
brother!), author and television writer and producer; and especially co-
author Meyer's daughter, Erica Meyer Rauzin, Miami Beach, Fla., former
editor of *South Florida* magazine, who found time while being a wife and
the mother of three of the Meyer grandchildren, to edit and organize this
book, and without whom it would never have been completed; and the
Meyer sons, writer David N. Meyer II, Ketchum, Idaho, a candid and
helpful critic, and Jason B. Meyer, Pennington, N.J., attorney and coun-
selor who guarded our legality in this new world of books and contracts.

We thank warmly the helpful volunteers who collected and collated
several hundred computer-printed pages, and our literary representative,
Herbert Schlosberg, Esq., of Los Angeles, Calif., whose good offices pro-
pelled us into the ranks of published authors.

Cy Nash and I express deep gratitude to the tolerant and painstaking people of the University of Chicago Press, among them our manuscript editor, Kathryn Krug. It was comforting to work with such a team in our first book-length venture.

Any errors, omissions, or misinterpretations in this book cannot be attributed to our gracious helpers and advisors but are solely the responsibility of the authors.

*   *   *

We thank also our wives, Sally Nash and Anne Meyer, for their forbearance during the long gestation and writing of this book and their advice, cautions, and criticisms as the chapters slowly emerged. This projected dominated their lives and controlled their schedules for what seems in retrospect a very long time. We appreciate them a great deal and, of course, have done so for additional reasons for many years.

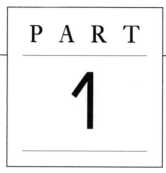

PART

1

1

Up in the Air to Ponder
What Could This Thing Be?

**I mulled, hopefully, over the nonmalignant possibilities
first, of course.**

I BEGAN TO STUDY the troubles the prostate can get into, both benign and
malignant, when it finally dawned on me I had a problem. Like many men,
I don't absorb bad news until I mull over it a bit. So I'd like to ease into this
part of the story with a little background.

Late in a warm Florida September, with my sixty-ninth birthday coming up in early October, my wife Anne and I returned to Miami from Walt
Disney World where we attended a reunion of the crew of my World War II
destroyer, the USS Foote (DD511). Almost fifty of the guys showed up,
not bad attendance considering the ship had been decommissioned some
forty-five years ago. The reunion offered a friendly, somewhat sentimental,
four-day reprisal of our youthful adventures in the South Pacific and paid a
memorial tribute to the men who had been killed in combat and those who
had died in the meantime.

We felt nice and warm about the reunion. The glow lingered as I buck-
led myself in the left seat of our six-place A36 Beechcraft Bonanza
(N9093Q) for the hour or so flight home. Anne sat in the co-pilot seat
ready to work the radios for me and pleased about the weather. She loves
flying, too, but not when the air is bumpy.

Flying has been an important part of our lives for more than forty years
since I took lessons under the World War II GI Bill. Every time I take off
and sense the ground falling away beneath me, I get a large charge of personal freedom that restores my feeling that liberation from traffic, bustling
crowds, and traffic signals really can be obtained, one way or the other.

I had passed my biennial FAA required Class 3 flight medical a couple
of weeks previously. The doctor chewed me out for still smoking and emphasized that smoking and flying at altitudes where the air's thin don't mix.
Smoke isn't good for the plane's instruments, either. I admit also that after

some fifty-five years of relatively light smoking—a pack a day—I theorized that if it were going to get me, stopping at this late stage wouldn't make much difference. But I wanted to quit if only to show myself I could.

Pushed by a tail wind and blessed by a sunny, clear day we breezed through the hundred and fifty miles to home in less than an hour, scooting pleasantly above central Florida's cattle-ranging plains and south Florida's endless fields of sugar cane, with the last fifteen minutes or so topping the Everglades. Just flying smoothly along made me look forward to an expected longer trip very soon to the Georgia hills where we had recently completed a mountain house, in the neighborhood of Gainesville, our home town before we moved to Miami in 1969. I wanted to plant some trees and shrubs that could only be transplanted in Georgia's fall or winter, and a brief trip northward beckoned. I didn't know as I lowered the Bonanza wheels and prepared to touch down at Opa-locka (sic) airport that except for one quick turn-around flight a Georgia excursion would be long delayed.

The next day I went through my annual physical with Dr. P. James Furlong, our family physician. EKG, lung x-ray, everything else checked out OK. He felt my prostate and said it seemed a little enlarged and advised me to see a urologist, Dr. Seymour Nash. This was the second time he suggested the referral, but I had managed to procrastinate. By the time of this exam, it was obvious I needed specialized attention. I was getting up four times a night to pee and infrequently felt some burning and pain.

Otherwise, I felt fine, was swimming regularly and playing a little golf with the usual frustrations. My normal sleep time for years has been slightly more than six hours but the frequent night calls (which I later learned are termed *nocturia*) were cutting into that extensively. I was wondering, too, what the urologist would find. I knew there were several problems possible with the prostate and its general system. I thought these caused more obvious symptoms, such as discharges or itching, pain, discomfort, burning urination. I could have an infection. I could have some venereal disease, though that was highly unlikely given my monogamous lifestyle.

Playing self-diagnostician, since I had no symptoms whatever, except for frequent urination, I ran through my remembered litany of possibilities and found I was left with (1) nothing but an old man's bladder, (2) non-malignant enlargement of the prostate, or (3) cancer of the prostate.

It was time for me to tend to my ailing anatomy, by actually visiting the doctor. I already knew enough to realize that no off-the-cuff diagnosis or instant treatment awaited.

I subscribe to a couple of excellent health newsletters, one from the

University of California at Berkeley and another from Harvard. They'd been paying considerable attention lately to the prostate and to assorted male urinary problems.

Maybe I had been too flip about all this. Maybe a lifetime of excellent health, to this point, had beguiled me. Not for the first time, it crossed my mind that perhaps I should have taken care of this earlier.

2

BPH and Other
Nonmalignant Problems
Maybe It's Just That We're Getting Older

A little knowledge means you think of the most optimistic result.

MY SYMPTOMS COULD HAVE BEEN CAUSED by several conditions other than cancer, the last thing I wanted to think about. In fact, it did not occur to me or to my wife Anne, who was all too aware of my frequent night prowls to the bathroom. She had been nudging me to see the doctor but thought, too, I had some routine trouble simply as a consequence of getting older.

I didn't discuss the possibilities with her, but I thought about them. What could I have developed?

For example: infections causing inflammation of the prostate, known as prostatitis; or *prostatodynia*, which means pain in the prostate (I had none); or enlargement of the prostate known as *benign prostatic hyperplasia* or BPH, the most common. It strikes about half of all men in their sixties.

In BPH the inner glands of the prostate enlarge. Their growth is somewhat checked by the outer tissues of the prostate, the capsule itself. This directs the enlargement inward and puts pressure on the urethra, which it surrounds, interfering with the flow of urine. The urethra carries urine from the bladder to the penis for discharge. Prostate enlargement can back up pressure against the bladder.

Changes in urination, such as my increased frequency, are the most prevalent symptoms. Other symptoms may include a delay in starting the stream, a tendency to dribble at the end, and incomplete emptying of the bladder. Men tend to strain when they have these problems, and such resistance thickens the bladder muscle giving a feeling of incomplete emptying. Involuntary spasms of that muscle occur, inducing a strong sense of urgency resulting in frequent trips to the bathroom to produce only small amounts of urine.

The pressure can lead to incontinence, and urination may become

6

uncontrollable. Or in its worst manifestation it can cause total urinary retention, meaning you cannot pee at all and require emergency medical attention. Extreme BPH can cause not only retention but stones, diverticula (protrusions of the inner lining of the bladder), blockage of the kidneys, and, in the end, uremic poisoning.

By far the most frequent treatment for BPH is *transurethral resection of the prostate*, known as TURP. This is a "coring out" of the prostate with instruments inserted through the urethra. It isn't a cancer cure. It relieves the pressure that enlarging prostate cells place on your urine voiding mechanism. You'll read more about it shortly because I went through the procedure. In the late nineteen-eighties, upwards of 300,000 TURPs were done in this country a year. More recently, newly developed and improved alternatives became available and the number of TURPs is declining.

Various drugs have been tried on BPH and experiments are being reported with "balloons"—small, elongated balloons inserted in the urethra and expanded with fluids to try to push enlarged tissues back in place. These are variants of the balloons used in angioplasty, a process that opens blockages of blood vessels serving the heart. Results appear to be short-run much of the time and the procedure has not become popular.

Some of the newer drugs have shown effectiveness against BPH. Proscar, the trade name for *finasteride*, can be helpful. It has been effective in about 30 percent of the cases in shrinking the prostate, but the statisticians are still keeping tabs on it. Proscar can take a long time, several months, to become effective.

Our co-author, Dr. Nash, has found Hytrin, trade name for *terazosin*, commonly used in treating high blood pressure, effective in about 50 percent of BPH cases. It is made by Abbott Laboratories. It relaxes the smooth muscles of the prostate and the bladder neck and decreases spasms, if any. Side effects are said to be minimal. One urologist among those who urged FDA approval for BPH treatment said he found close to 80 percent of the men using Hytrin got effective relief from enlargement symptoms within two or three weeks.

Both drugs were recently approved by the Food and Drug Administration for widespread use. Proscar's manufacturer, Merck and Co., is providing daily pills for some eighteen thousand men, half of whom will receive Proscar and half a placebo over a seven-year period to see if it is effective as a preventative for prostate cancer, since it affects the action of male hormones on the prostate and hormones influence the growth of prostate cancer cells. Depriving the male body of the male hormone, testosterone, is a standard treatment for advanced prostate cancer. Other drugs are more effective for that purpose once cancer has advanced, but they can cause impotence and other problems. Current knowledge—the tests may prove otherwise—holds that 4 percent of Proscar users may have potency problems, perhaps with ejaculation. The pill must be taken daily for life by men on whom it proves effective.

It takes a long time for changes in treatment to be proven, but the scope of the Proscar tests assures high statistical veracity when the tests are concluded. Even if Proscar or Hytrin relieves only 30 percent of the U.S. men with prostatic enlargement they could prevent more than 100,000 of the annual surgical procedures currently being applied to the problem in this country.[1]

BPH affects literally hundreds of thousands of men each year and many do not want, or are not in good enough health for, an operation. So the search for other options in treatment, in addition to drugs, continues. Some of these are fairly new and so will require time and an accumulation of patient histories to test their usefulness. Procedures drawing professional attention include the following:

"Stents": A stent is a tubular net that looks remotely like the Chinese finger lock puzzle that captures fingers inserted at each end. The stent is smaller, of course, and is placed in the urethra to maintain openness. Use of these options rests on the situation in each individual case, but stents seem primarily used for older men.

Heat: Technically called *transurethral microwave therapy,* this process uses a catheter through the penis to apply heat to the prostate. Special instruments provide simultaneous cooling for adjacent areas that shouldn't be heated.

Laser: With the acronym TULIP, *transurethral ultrasound-guided laser-induced prostatectomy* is under testing by the Food and Drug Administration and holds promise for quick and bloodless treatment.

Laser: *visual ablation* differs from TULIP in the manner of laser application. Doctors involved in trials said the process appears to be effective with fewer aftereffects and lower costs than a TURP.

Incision of the prostate: a transurethral procedure less invasive than a TURP for especially selected patients and those who are "medically unstable" and should not risk the more invasive TURP operation.

If laser surgery meets the expectations of its practitioners it still will confront a major urological concern: neither the procedure nor the medical treatments (drugs) provide tissue for pathological examination and so the cancer that occurs in about 10 percent of BPH cases will not be discovered as it would be in a TURP. Not to worry, says Dr. John N. Kabalin of Stanford, "it is a bit fortuitous that we have seen the parallel development [along with non-invasive therapies] of diagnostic technologies, such as PSA [prostatic specific antigen blood test] and ultrasound-guided biopsies, that may more than make up for this lack of a pathological specimen related to treatment."[2]

Currently, however, the TURP still represents important treatment to a lot of guys who've been getting up several times a night to pee, dribbling in their jockey shorts during the day, and otherwise being besieged. You see them all the time behind the trees on the golf course.

I didn't know it at the time, but I had some BPH along with my prostate cancer and was retaining about 400 cc (about 13 fluid ounces) of urine that was not being voided; I was completely surprised later when Dr. Nash found that little reservoir in my bladder, so I underwent a TURP. It is a full-fledged surgical procedure and in my case was quite effective and more annoying than painful.

Stephen N. Rous, M.D., in *The Prostate Book,* distributed by the Consumers Union, examines benign prostatic hyperplasia in exhaustive detail, emphasizing the dangers involved in retention of urine, caused by pressure from the enlarged prostate on the bladder. Once retention starts, he writes, it tends to increase and can lead to infection, blood in the urine, and formation of stones in the bladder. These are sneaky problems because they advance slowly and the man gets sort of used to them, delaying his visit to his doctor.

If cancer can be diagnosed before a TURP is undertaken for BPH, and if total removal of the prostate (radical prostatectomy) is indicated for the cancer, it will not be necessary to have two operations, because with the prostate gone, the BPH will of course be gone, too.

Dr. Rous noted that patients treated successfully for BPH experience a dramatic improvement and feel better than they have in a long time. That was certainly true in my case, but we're concentrating more on prostate cancer in this book and will not examine other prostate problems in detail, except to let you know they exist and alert you to the necessity of treatment.

Though prostatic enlargement is called "benign" (simply because it is not malignant) BPH is nothing to fool around with. Sometimes, when a TURP or other therapy is not indicated, an open incision is made and the enlarged "pulp" of the prostate interior is removed through operations known as suprapubic or retropubic subtotal prostatectomy.

We're talking here about removal of perhaps a quantity of tissue the size of a lemon, or in cases of large prostates, an orange or an apple. An open subtotal might be called for if the prostate is very large, or the doctor needs to cut out some diverticula or remove several stones not subject to lithotripsy (crushing them with sound waves), lasers, or other noninvasive techniques. These procedures aren't as common as TURPs but they accomplish the same thing. Dr. Nash notes that every surgeon has his own limit regarding the size of a prostate he is willing to subject to a TURP. All surgeons aren't trained the same and an oversize prostate could present some difficulties to a doctor not accustomed to treating them with a TURP.

Discovery of cancer in tissue from a TURP or from an open prostatectomy is a signal for probable further treatment. The TURP is not a cure for cancer since it rarely removes all the tissues inside the prostatic capsule. Also, the shell, or the capsule—you might say the "rind"—remains intact. Many men live for years with some leftover microscopic evidences of cancer from their TURP. You may read in some reports of concern that a TURP might release cancerous cells into the bloodstream and help spread the cancer. More recent studies refute this assertion but the National Cancer Institute's *PDQ* publication, regularly distributed as a periodic update for physicians, continues to publish a cautionary statement.

Another benign prostate problem is prostatitis, inflammation of the prostate, which comes in three varieties: acute bacterial prostatitis, chronic bacterial prostatitis, and nonbacterial prostatitis. The latter is the most common and mostly strikes men from thirty to fifty years old. It is painful and is called *prostatodynia,* meaning prostatic pain. What causes it isn't known precisely but usually it is considered to be stress-related, probably from chronic tension of the pelvic floor muscles. Effective treatment is difficult. Chronic prostatitis may lie dormant for a long time but when it flares the symptoms can include pain in the testicles, burning urination, and, some of my earlier sources have written, changes in sexual desire (both increased and decreased), and perhaps some discharge and backache following sexual intercourse. There is disagreement on the latter symptoms, but if you experience them see your urologist.

Nonbacterial prostatitis frequently is nothing more nor less than an accumulation of fluids in the prostate due to insufficient ejaculation, although a urologist-advisor isn't sure this is true, either. In any event, others believe restoring the usual pattern of intercourse or masturbation brings relief. Not all urologists agree with Dr. Monroe Greenberger[3] that this is one of the more pleasant prescriptions for a patient available to a urologist. Neither do they agree about repeated prostate massage through the rectum by the doctor's finger. One said more than three or four massages are unnecessary except to the physician's income, unless the patient is unable to have intercourse or is emotionally incapable of masturbation. Greenberger recommends massage, especially for younger men who've enjoyed a frustrating interlude with an only partially cooperative viz-à-viz.[4]

So, briefly, these were troubles I might have had—though we already know, except for a slight BPH problem, I was headed for the concern I didn't want to think about. I would have welcomed a prescription ordering me to hurry and get more sex.

There's a favorite story in northern Georgia about a doctor, now deceased, who was asked by a patient, "Dr. Ben, how old should a man be when he stops masturbating?" "I don't know," Ben replied. "I'm forty-five. You'll have to ask an older doctor than me."[5]

Here Comes the Finger

Doctor's Suspicions Aroused

Most doctors recognize that medicine is just as much an art
as it is a science and that the most important knowledge in
medicine to be learned or taught is the way the human body can
summon innermost resources to meet extraordinary challenges.
NORMAN COUSINS, *Anatomy of an Illness*

WHEN I FIRST MET Seymour Nash, M.D., F.A.C.S., I sensed I would come
to know him well and that we would be associated for a long time. Whatever
had attacked me would not be repulsed in a week or two, like a bad cold.
Nash was a trim, pleasantly smiling, and crisply businesslike person in his
white doctor's coat. He moved as though he had no time to waste and, indeed, he did not, since glum looking people occupied every chair in his
waiting room.

Our brief introductory conversation revealed that we were fraternity
brothers. His chapter was at the University of Florida and mine at the University of North Carolina. I would not make too much of fraternalism forty
or so years after college but there is a mutually recognizable bond. At least,
I thought facetiously, he'd better take good care of me or I would report
him to headquarters.

I perceived, also, that while he would willingly answer any question I
asked, his presumption—quite accurate, of course—was that, like most
new patients, I didn't know enough to understand any brief fill-ins from
him, and he did not have time to review medicology from *Gray's Anatomy* to
the present. Later, when I had educated myself somewhat and he agreed to
collaborate with me on this book, we set up special times for "literary" discussions and on regular visits I stuck strictly to my patient's role.

My initial visit went quickly. I bent over a table and he stuck his finger
in my rear end. It was unpleasant but it didn't hurt. I felt he was reaching
for my back teeth but knew his finger was only so long and he didn't have to
reach far, only about two inches. This exam was my introduction to pros-

tate disease's invasive nature and its ignorance of the usual standards of privacy. If you have some reluctance to have strangers diddling about hitherto intimate areas of your body, forget it. Modesty is not part of the therapy.

In his office after the exam, Cy was brief and to the point. "Felt some lumps in your prostate and perhaps at least one on the outside of the prostate. Very suspicious. You may have prostate cancer. But I want to do some more tests."

In the movies, this is where the patient asks, "How long have I got?" or gives some other indication of appreciation of the gravity of the judgment. When Nash said he wanted more tests, he obviously wasn't ready for neat definitions of my problem.

He probably thought I was stunned into silence. Perhaps I was, but I recall no conscious reaction whatever. I wasn't numb; I just didn't react, almost as though he were talking about someone else. Maybe I thought his further tests would prove him wrong, because how could I have cancer and not hurt somewhere? I said nothing.

He said, "I felt only a slight enlargement of your prostate. It may be that the cancer is pressing on the urethra and causing the frequent urination. We'll have to see."

He took blood to send to a lab for a prostatic specific antigen (PSA) assay. PSA is the fairly new procedure that measures a substance secreted by a troubled prostate gland. The test significantly advanced prostate cancer discovery and management.

Two days later, we met at Mt. Sinai Medical Center on Miami Beach, a major hospital that also works with Jackson Memorial Hospital of Miami (University of Miami Medical School) in teaching and is part of the South Florida Comprehensive Cancer Center network. Plenty of expertise around if needed, I felt, but the more I saw of Cy Nash and his work the less I wanted to get involved with other medical advisors at this stage. Nevertheless, a second opinion on something this serious is a good idea unless you have absolute confidence in your primary urologist. Some insurance companies may require a second evaluation.

Washington Post staffer Hobart Rowen in early 1992 presented an urgent reason for seeking a second opinion. He was diagnosed at Georgetown Hospital in Washington with a bladder cancer and was placed on intravenous chemical therapy using an especially powerful chemical. Through a series of glitches and a delayed report, it was some twenty days later he was informed that he had, not bladder cancer, but prostate cancer. Then, he says, "I took my cancer in my own hands," and went to Johns Hopkins in Baltimore. The prostate cancer was confirmed and he was put on medication to stop his body's use of the male hormone testosterone which fuels the cancer. I talked with him after his article strongly advocating second opinions was published in the *Post* and by that time he was feeling well, but still angry about his original diagnosis.

In my newspaper and magazine days I served on a citizens' health facility review board and so I knew the local medical community and some members of the University of Miami medical staff well enough to inquire about Nash. They thought highly of him.

I passed on a second opinion but that ancient joke ran through my mind: The patient says, "I want a second opinion." "OK," says the doctor, "You're ugly, too."

Further Anatomical Probing

Cy told me my PSA test yielded a score of 14, a level almost certainly indicative of cancer. I had this to mull over during the rest of the process. He would explain the PSA in more detail later.

Cy had me lie on my side on an examining table. It occurred to me, not for the first time, that these tables must be deliberately designed so narrow as to leave your arms unsupported and force you to dangle them or hug yourself or strain not to dangle. This may be kind of an automatic stress test to keep patients humble.

As I lay there, I could see a monitor, like a gray television screen. Cy intruded an ultrasound probe into my now further humiliated body. The screen before me swirled with gray and dark gray blotches broken by irregular patches of lighter gray. What I saw would not be significant to me, Cy said. Later I would see pictures of ultrasound probing in medical books and even with briefings could differentiate very little, even when the pictures were labeled with arrows and numbers. For fifteen minutes or so he moved the probe around. With his instruments he could see in there and he could also see the screen, from which he was printing out pictures all the while.

Associated with the probe was a small machine that stuck fine needles through the rectum wall into the prostate area. This was a Biopty gun. The needles withdrew tissue samples for later laboratory analysis. I could hear the needle device click and when it did I felt a little thump, like a finger snap. Except for the discomfort of the invading probe I felt no pain. Cy worked with dispatch, no comments, no conversation, not even a medical "hmm."[1]

While the ultrasound screen further confirmed Nash's earlier judgment that cancer was present, its primary purpose was to help him aim the needle that extracted the tissues. The tissues would be examined by pathologists to diagnose and define the pattern of the cancer cells and to analyze them to determine their precise condition, aggressiveness, and structure. This is *histology*, the study of cells. These finer definitions would provide some guide to treatment and would help "grade" the cancer. This was my first introduction to prostate cancer grading, known as the Gleason grade.

Staging defines the location and the extent of the cancer. *Grading* defines the nature of the cancer cells themselves, dealing with the possible aggressiveness of the cells and other information that can be read from their microscopic appearance.[2]

The next day I went to a local radiology office, duly signed the standard disclaimer forms and endured a full drill of tests at the hands of apparently competent people who launched their work immediately and impersonally. They took a range of xrays and did an intravenous pyelogram (IVP). That is, they injected a dye—more accurately, a "contrast medium"—in my arm. This is an iodinated compound that improves the xray look into the bladder, kidneys, and other assorted organs and pipes. It nauseated me immediately. I threw up a little and then felt OK. They hastened to tell me this doesn't happen to everyone. That's true. My reaction was unusual.

There is another form of the medium, *nonionic*, which produces even fewer side reactions but costs about ten times as much as the "older" contrast. Some places use it exclusively, some only for high-risk patients. There was an estimate a couple of years ago that if all IVP exams switched to nonionic contrasts it would add a billion dollars a year to the cost of medical care in this country. However, if anyone had bothered to explain the difference in reactions to me in advance I'd gladly have paid my share.

The xrays covered me from the upper abdomen down through the lower pelvic area looking for spread of cancer, bone involvement, bladder condition, and other anomalies. This was a two-hour exercise. In a brief chat with Cy, after he'd seen the tests, I learned I was carrying about 13 ounces of fluid in my bladder and that would make further treatment difficult if we were to use radiation therapy against the cancer. We would have to get rid of that fluid and restore a more normal urination schedule.

To achieve that happy state, I learned, I would need a TURP. All I knew about it was what I'd heard in uninformed conversation roughly of the intellectual level of nine-year-old boys discussing sex. I kept referring to the procedure as the "rotor-rooter" operation. The doctors didn't think that was funny and, besides, it was quite wrong because the surgeon does not use a "rooter" at all. He uses a small instrument that employs a tiny wire loop along with a scope that enables him to see inside. He uses foot pedals to control the wire either for removing tissue or for cauterizing wounds, preventing bleeding. Eventually, the urethra relines itself. Cy felt now that the blockage was caused by cancer, but that there was some BPH (enlargement of the prostate) influence, also. Something else to think about.

Now, the decision for treatment of my probable cancer between radiation or a radical prostatectomy, meaning surgery, was bearing down on me. I didn't yet know how to make the decision or what factors were involved in it.

Cy explained that I would need a TURP before radiation, because once I started treatment, if I went into urinary retention and required a catheter to void, the treatment would have to be interrupted or delayed, not good practice, as it would reduce the effectiveness of the radiation. He also explained that if I chose the surgical route, a TURP would not be necessary, as the entire prostate would be removed, anyway.

I was leaning toward radiation and without realizing it, was breaking my own rule by moving toward a decision insufficiently informed. I really didn't fully understand all the options at that time. The final decision would come later, after more tests and scans.

I did hear a phrase I would see and hear again in the course of handling this disease: It's your decision.

When the Two-By-Four Hits You
The Symptoms, If Any at All

Carcinoma of the prostate is predominantly a tumor
of older men, which frequently responds to treatment even
when widespread and may be cured when localized. The rate of
tumor growth varies from moderately rapid to very slow, and
patients may live five years or more even after the cancer has
metastasized. Since the median age at diagnosis is 70 years [the
average age is 73] many patients, especially those with localized
tumor, may die of other illnesses without ever having
suffered significant disability from their cancer.
from the National Cancer Institute's *PDQ State of the Art* cancer treatment
periodic information bulletin

THE PDQ BULLETIN is published for doctors. Its cover paragraph (above) struck me as one of the more cheerful statements I confronted in medical literature. But it failed to answer my more urgent questions. Would this invader kill me and if so when? How fast would my personal tumor grow if not stopped? Was it the kind that would start growths (metastasize) beyond the prostate gland if it was still confined to that gland (localized)? How fast would it grow? Was there anything I could eat or drink that might make it go away, or at least not spread? Why did 25 to 33 percent of the men who get it die in time and others live? And more.

None of the books aimed at the lay victim really answered those questions. Waiting for my transurethral resection—the TURP—I began my self-education by reading: the books and booklets of the American Cancer Society, relevant articles from medical journals, especially urological journals obtained from the University of Miami Medical School library, special papers and journals from various physicians' meetings here and abroad.

Indeed, having committed to the TURP was in fact a commitment to radiation, as well. Cy Nash would tell me later that radiation was my better choice.

Friends, including other members of my growing informal prostate cancer (PCa)[1] alliance, sent me copies of booklets issued by their doctors and hospitals. Some were quite good, with informative detail in broad terms about what the patient might expect. None answered the fundamental questions piling up in my head. They did tell me about treatment options but made no comparisons or judgments. Few prepared me to ask relevant questions of my doctor.

I found more statistics in American Cancer Society and National Cancer Institute publications than I could absorb, compilations of figures on how many patients lived how long after which treatment, broken down into various categories according to the extent of their cancers when discovered, their ages when diagnosed, the time span before recurrence if any, and more. As I read, I began to fall into the vernacular used by the doctors and researchers in the field as their terms on this subject sank into my spongy brain cells. I resolved, as a reporter, to put their lingo into lay terms for the general reader.

Most prostate cancers remain asymptomatic, that is, causing no outward symptoms or even minor pain, for a very long time. Yet, four thousand more cases will be discovered in men each year than cases of lung cancer. Dr. Howard Scher of the Memorial Sloan-Kettering Center, New York, wrote in *Current Opinion in Oncology* (1991) that by the year 2000, a 90 percent increase in annual incidence and a 37 percent increase in annual mortality are projected. The statisticians tallied 165,000 cases in 1993, up from 135,000 in 1992, and expect 200,000 cases and 38,000 deaths in 1994.

Internists or family practitioners suspect some of these cancers and refer patients to urologists, although urologists believe referrals because of digital rectal exams amount to only a minor fraction of discoveries. Cy Nash urges men to go to a urologist with experience. "You don't go to a dentist for your heart," he says. "No one can be expert at everything in medicine and there've been a lot of changes in urology, especially."

You'll find if you ask, that doctors other than urologists think they are quite capable of doing a sound digital exam although they concede, as "presumption," one of my informal advisors told me, that urologists' experience means the specialists might miss fewer tumors.

With the advent of the prostatic specific antigen (PSA) blood test procedure, however, more internists and general practitioners are finding suspicious readings resulting in more and earlier referrals. The increase in cancers discovered can in large part be attributed to the PSA. This also means discovery of more early, or prostate confined, tumors. In time, it could reduce death rates because still-confined tumors may be cured. More years must pass before tomorrow's mortality tables reflect today's advanced technology.

Yet the large number of prostate cancer diagnoses forms the crux of a major current debate in urology concerning whether all found should be treated. We'll get into this in part 2 of this book.

Don't assume your own internist thoroughly understands the significance of the PSA. A friend, now in his mid-seventies, routinely received a clean bill from his family doctor over several years of digital rectal exams. Last year he asked the doctor, "What's this PSA test I've read about?" The doctor replied, "If you want one, I'll give it to you."

My friend, a former newspaper colleague and one of the nation's leading advertising sales executives, then learned to his dismay that his PSA reading was 110. (Mine, you'll recall, had been 14.) He discovered that he was carrying a metastasized prostate cancer, stage D2. Bone scans showed two metastases with suspicious indications of a third. He was seriously ill yet he had never felt a twinge of pain. His disease had advanced beyond surgery or radiation therapy. He immediately began taking hormone-suppressing drugs. A year after the diagnosis we played a round of golf together. He felt fine and hit the ball well. But we both knew he'd be lucky to be among the 20 percent with his problem who would die in good time of something else.

It was a family practitioner digital rectal exam (DRE) referral, however, that led to a finding of PCa in a former shipmate of mine, a man I hadn't seen for thirty-five years. He heard through the ship's alumni grapevine that I was studying prostate cancer and called to tell me his cancer was discovered just that way. He'd never felt pain nor had a symptom of any kind. His PSA was a low normal 2.2. This seemed a discrepancy to me but I learned that in somewhere between 17 and 30 percent of the cases of prostate cancer the PSA will be normal. Such broad ranges in statistics are common in this disease. He enjoyed marathon running and even that strenuous exercise had caused no pain except a few muscle aches from time to time. The presence of the cancer was verified by ultrasound and a biopsy.[2]

So, How Do You Know?

Cancer symptoms might include frequency of urination, blood in the semen, difficulty in urination or even retention of urine. They might include bone pain or lower back pain.

For emphasis, let's list the possible symptoms. Remember, you may have none at all:

—need to urinate frequently, especially to awaken in the night several times (nocturia)

—a weak or interrupted flow

—blood in the urine or semen

—urine flow you can't easily stop

—burning or pain while urinating

—continuous pain in the pelvis, upper thighs, or lower back (these can occur even when there are no urination problems)

By the time the cancer causes pain anywhere, it may have progressed beyond a curable stage, though it certainly can, and must, be treated. This is why early discovery, before those bad cells can spread outside the prostate, is critical. If you stick to your trusted family physician, make sure he does a PSA test every year.

The best counsel, however, is that men over forty have a rectal exam every year, by a trained urologist. Good as your family internist may be, he may not find an early cancer. The urologist will take a blood sample for a PSA test. He'll do a digital rectal exam and maybe a transrectal ultrasound exam and a biopsy if your PSA is elevated or the DRE raises suspicions. In the recent past, biopsies were so painful as to require anesthesia but now, with the fast, fine needle Biopty gun, they are a minor annoyance. A biopsy provides tissues for microscopic exams and definitive proof that cancer is present. Unfortunately, a negative biopsy doesn't always prove cancer is not present.

*   *   *

I finally did the sensible thing and visited Dr. Nash when I could sleep no longer than twenty minutes at a stretch without having to stumble my way to the bathroom. Frequently, I'd sleep for only fifteen minutes before awakening again. I had no pain, no burning, no incontinence in the daytime, but I was stupid to put up with the nuisance as long as I did. Indeed, I may have been lucky in a way that the cancer and BPH put pressure on my urethra and alerted me. Otherwise, it would have had time to get worse. So, seek the tests, including the exploratory finger.

Early in my research, the working title of this book was "Up Yours!" It was intended as an admonition and an urgent plea. On second thought, it sounded somewhat flip and perhaps pejorative, so we abandoned it. But the advisory meaning should be clear to you by now. Spread the word.

What the Exams Are Like
Meet the Searching Machines

Despite the barium cocktail and the apprehension about machine-induced claustrophobia, I survived the second round of anatomical investigations.

NOW I WAS DOUBLY ANXIOUS to get up to the Georgia hills to take care of some house chores and to confer with one Charles Marvin Silverstein, M.D., F.A.C.R., of Atlanta, about fifty-five miles from the mountain house we call "The Peak."

Marvin (called "Charles" by a few of his Atlanta colleagues) and I have known each other since we were about two years old and have remained close all these years. In fact, Marvin had early ambitions to be a journalist also and was graduated from Emory University with a degree in journalism. He decided, however, that he wanted to be a doctor and studied medicine at Emory.

Back in the olden days, I worked one summer as a reporter-intern at the *Atlanta Journal*. Marvin was a senior med student. I would join him Saturday nights at Grady Hospital, part of my "beat" for the paper, don a white coat, and hang around the emergency room looking for stories. At "the Gradys," Atlanta's giant public and teaching hospital, in the course of a Saturday night just about every trauma known to science would appear. And more on nights of a full moon!

A radiologist, Marvin was one of the founding physicians of Northside Hospital in Atlanta. Over the years it, too, grew into a major medical center along with the city's exploding northside suburbs. I wanted Marvin to supervise my further tests—bone scans, a CT ("cat" or Computerized Tomography) scan and possibly an MRI (Magnetic Resonance Imaging) scan if Marvin thought that necessary. The other tests indicated it wasn't.[1]

So, my then-seven-year-old granddaughter Dara and I strapped ourselves into the Bonanza and took off in an unusually cloudless sky for north Georgia. Private flying is just another means of transportation to Dara.

One of her little friends spoke of a trip with her grandfather and Dara asked, "What kind of an airplane does he fly?"

Three and a half hours later we landed at Gainesville's Lee Gilmer Memorial Airport, were picked up, and in a half hour more were on The Peak surveying 220 degrees of mountain scenery. I remember thinking then of the cancer growing somewhere behind my pubic bone and that it would be a particularly bitter fate if I were to be denied extensive enjoyment of this retreat in the geography I loved so much.

A day or so later, Marvin drove up to The Peak, bringing some pamphlets about prostate cancer. We had a serious discussion of my problem. He described it as not good but not as bad as I might be afraid. He had talked with Nash and agreed, before seeing the additional test results, that my cancer stage was probably a B2, maybe bordering on a C, as Nash's finger exam suggested possible involvement of the seminal vesicles, which are alongside the prostate, meaning there might be some tumor outside the prostate capsule itself.

Marvin was reassuring but not patronizing. He said this is my cancer and I must take charge of it and not let anyone do anything with it I didn't understand and agree with.

This was key advice all cancer patients should observe. I want to emphasize it. Make sure you understand every step of your examinations and treatments. Stop the process if you are unsure.

Marvin set me up for the Northside procedures the following Tuesday. Marvin would report the results to Nash. This was a Friday. I would spend Monday night at his house to be near the hospital for 7:10 a.m. tests. In the meantime, I wanted to start my education in earnest.

I began with dinner with Carl Lawson and his wife, Ginny. Our friendship goes way back to the earliest of my twenty-two years in Gainesville, nineteen of them as editor of the *Times*, which I joined as a reporter three days before it began daily publication January 26, 1947. Carl had recently completed an apparently successful series of radiation treatments for his prostate cancer.

His was discovered early and almost by accident. He had some urethral blockage but no cancer was suspected. His TURP tissue biopsy showed some cancer, a finding in about one in ten TURP procedures. It appeared totally confined to the prostate. Carl took twenty-seven daily radiation zaps, did his routine jogging of two miles or so every morning after treatment and felt fine. He has always been in good physical condition. He is a nonsmoker, and although no relation between smoking and prostate cancer has been identified, one's general health is important to handling this intruder. The talk with Carl was comforting. The details of his exams and of the radiation treatment, which I knew I had coming, started that familiarity with the process that helps build one's confidence.

Nevertheless, I knew my cancer was worse than his. Nash's tentative classification of a B2/C (he had not seen the CT results) confirmed that. A classification of C or D is threatening. It means there is cancerous tissue beyond the prostate capsule—extending perhaps into lymph nodes or bone. Doctors feel that cancer that extends beyond the prostate may not be curable by radiation or surgery but may be by cryosurgery (freezing) which can reach slightly beyond the prostate capsule to where a stage C cancer may lurk. Not all agree. Some state flatly that a cancer extending beyond the capsule is not curable.

Certainly they didn't mean it is not treatable or stoppable, at least for a time. They don't say what they mean by "curable." Do they mean the cancer will kill me immediately? Obviously not. Even men with advanced cases may take two to five years, some far longer, to succumb. Will the cancer progressively invade other organs, the lymph system, the pelvic bones, leading to slow and painful debilitation and death? If it can't be stopped it may do just that. Cy Nash feels that to consider a patient cured, fifteen years must pass with no evidence of recurring disease. However, if you make five years after initial treatment your chances of longer survival improve significantly.

Carl's experience, while not happy, seemed relatively mild since his cancer was caught in a timely manner. Carl's story calmed me somewhat, countering the suspicion that I could die of this stuff before my expected time, perhaps even within two or three years if it could not be controlled.

I also began to be impressed with the fact that I was facing miserable treatments, at the very least, and a real shift in my personal timetables for writing, enjoying my new house and my grandkids, and even flying a lot now that I was retired from those forty-plus years of twelve- and fourteen-hour work days, all to be confronted in this, the month of my sixty-ninth birthday. One problem, of course, is that it is difficult to wipe your mind clean of this internal contamination and, like the "automatic engine rough" you hear when flying a single engine plane over long stretches of water, every little muscle and nerve twinge evoked the spook in my insides. You learn to ignore these irrelevant signals. Cancer pain is constant. You'll know it's not a passing flash.

In truth, I wasn't afraid of dying nor did I worry about death, except for my eternally unsatisfied curiosity. It is true that as you approach advanced age, though you still feel young inside, you realize immortality is not for humans and slowly adjust to reality. Besides—and if this sounds melodramatic, forgive me—my combat experience in World War II, while not as intense nor prolonged as many other sailors', sufficed. My first kamikaze attack, in the Philippines, acted as a catharsis of terror, enough to allow me in subsequent incidents to suppress fear and function as I was supposed to. However, I cannot suppress an inner awareness that since those days I have been living on borrowed time, anyway. I find many other combat veterans have that feeling.

What's It Like to Go through the Scans?

The night before the Northside tests Marvin had me drink fourteen ounces of barium in an orange-flavored sherbert, in preparation for the various scans upcoming. The barium sank like concrete in my insides and throughout the night exerted pressure on some unidentifiable sensitive points, causing numerous trips to the john. My longest sleep stretch was about forty-five minutes after an initial ninety minute snooze.

Finally, morning came and I had some cantaloupe and coffee and set off to the hospital, trying to track Marvin's car through a damp, dark morning on a four-lane highway carrying what eight lanes of traffic couldn't have handled. I lost him, of course.

"You're a great doctor, Silverstein," I muttered to myself, "but don't you ever look in your rearview mirror?"

I fumbled around exits and entrances until I located the parking lot he had designated. This delay triggered my anxiety reflexes, but unnecessarily, as it turned out, because the check-in lady had just set up shop.

It triggered my voiding reflexes, also.

I barely started the check-in process when I had an immediate and urgent need to pee, plus pressure on the bowels. Someone occupied the nearest facility and I denounced him and all his kinfolks (to myself) and scurried to another one, but just as I entered the door was disastrously incontinent, front and rear, soaking my underwear but fortunately not my pants. I cleaned myself up and threw my underwear into a plastic trash bag.

This was my first experience with incontinence and it taught me not to delay when the first urge strikes. Later, on Cy Nash's advice, I would attend the john at least every couple of hours whether I needed to or not. I carry a "Little John," a plastic bottle, in the airplane for flights long or short and now carry it in my car, as well. I spent the rest of the time at Northside Hospital sans underwear, and very conscious of that fact, but no one checked up on me. I got away with it.

Preparing for the CT scan, I received an injection of dye and more barium. No reaction. I dreaded the CT scan because the pictures of the machine I had seen made the scanner look like a deep, small-bore tunnel that would overwhelm me with claustrophobia and in a prolonged exam would have me screaming for space.

That was also a misapprehension. The scanner is more like a doughnut with a thickness of eighteen inches or so, and you are not completely ingested by it, as I feared. Your head goes through and comes out the other side. Again, you climb onto a narrow table which moves you automatically through the scanning ring as xrays fire in sequence, reporting to a computer that turns the information into dimensional pictures. This machine bore a General Electric logo. It was seven or eight feet tall, a big shell of some white plastic material presiding over the extended table. I learned later that most of the real works of the machine, an arrangement of boxes, coils, and wires taller than my head (I'm six-two) and too big for a pickup truck, are in an adjacent shielded room.

The sharply defined pictures fabricated by the computer are more like detailed black-and-white drawings than xray photos. Each represents a cross-section of your body, as though you had been neatly sliced through. Even to the uneducated eye, the organs, bones, and spaces in the body are recognizable and easily distinguished. The pictures are amazingly graphic and clear. After the CT exam, other scans were made of my bones which showed in sharp relief against the now dispersed dye. All the technicians worked swiftly and efficiently, were helpful and friendly and avoided comments of any kind. They do not interpret: that's a doctor's job. They are also totally impersonal. You could be wearing a loin cloth and a necklace of bear's teeth or you could be naked as a jay bird and I don't think they'd notice.

As you expect in a hospital, everyone except the patient is interrupted from time to time and goes off to do something else, God knows what. Probably they go to another task which, like the one you are involved in, is interrupted also, leaving for these people as the day goes by a whole array of serially interrupted chores that by day's end must somehow be completed. Not easy.

With the pictures clipped to a large vertical light screen before him, one of Marvin's colleagues, Dr. Robert Tyrrel, guided me through his interpretations of the tests. Remarkably, even I could identify the cross-sections of most of the assorted organs pictured. The doctor said he found no indication whatsoever of any spread of the cancer beyond the prostate: not in bone, lymph glands, or elsewhere. The bone scan showed nothing, either.

"At first," Dr. Tyrrel said, "I saw something suspicious, but it turned out to be merely some arthritic bone growth. There's nothing to indicate months or years of a spread from a prostatic source."

This was good news, of course, and was reported back to Dr. Nash and to the whole family who were glad to have some upbeat news. The process was tedious but worth it. It did not mean there was no cancer in or immediately outside the prostate as the CT scan doesn't see into glands very well. The tests suggested a stage B2 cancer, but there was still enough doubt to maintain the possibility of a C. I would keep the slash and stay a B2/C. The radiologists stressed that when x-ray film or CT scan film and the urologist in charge do not agree, the priority interpretation goes with the physician's digital exam finding. His educated finger ranks above all the hi-tech probing. It remains true even though that finger cannot reach a substantial area of the prostate.

So, though the new tests were encouraging, I knew enough by now (I read a lot) to confirm in my mind that I would not have a radical prostatectomy in which my prostate would be removed by surgery. Dr. Nash's suspicious finger finding that bump on or right under the surface of the capsule argued in my mind for radiation. I knew, too, that Dr. Nash would not agree to radiation if he did not think it the advisable course of action. Surgery is usually reserved for A and B stage tumors that by definition are confined entirely within the prostate gland, although depending on the patient's general health, surgery may sometimes be used for stage C cancer, frequently to be followed by radiation or hormonal blockade. Also, hormonal blockade may be used prior to surgery in an attempt to "downstage" the tumor. More than one therapeutic mode may be used in a treatment regimen. We'll see that as we go through the various modes in detail.

Surgery is thought to be more curative when the cancer is totally within the prostate since no prostatic tissue remains in which the cancer can recur after the operation. Whether long-term clinical results of cures of A and B stages are about the same with radiation treatment remains a controversial matter. We think the surgical argument for truly capsule-confined tumors is gaining ground in newer studies.[2]

The decision for external beam radiation grew firmer. I don't like being rendered unconscious and I dreaded the hospitalization and the extended recovery interval following surgery. And if, indeed, there was some microscopic extension of the cancer cells radiation might subdue them.

Little did I realize at that time that the upcoming TURP would knock me out completely and also require a few days in that place where they take well people and make them sick.

Now, if the fall thundershowers let up, I'd fly out of the hills (it was going to get cold soon in the mountains, anyway) and make like a big white bird back to Florida. There I would have the TURP, a week or so in the hospital, and then on to whatever else Cy Nash and his cohorts had in store for me.

6

A Pigeonhole Just for You
What It Means to Be Graded and Staged

**Let's start with finding out who is sick and who is not.
My feeling is that the most important thing you confront in private
practice is when a man comes to you and wants to know whether
he has cancer of the prostate. That's the first thing to determine.**
SEYMOUR C. NASH, M.D.

JUST HOW SICK WAS I? Nothing hurt. I felt fine. Where on the scale of little cancers to big cancers, indolent cancers to raging cancers, did mine fit?

Once your urologist determines there's prostate cancer present, his diagnosis moves to a different level. Treatment will depend on specific knowledge of your cancer. Your cancer now must be "staged" and "graded." As I talked with dozens of prostate cancer patients I was surprised that many did not know the stage and grade of their problem. This would be like not knowing whether you had a bad cold or double pneumonia.

Determining whether cancer is present and categorizing it according to universally standard grading and staging systems are to an extent concurrent processes. Broadly described, *staging* classifies the location and spread, if any, of the cancer. *Grading* classifies the pathology of the cancer cells, that is, it attempts to rank the status, virulence, and possible growth rate of the tumor itself.

Your stage and grade become items of utmost importance to you. To a considerable extent, they will determine what treatment you may need. Each of the various stages, plus your general health and age, suggests possible differences in therapies. As you read about prostate cancer, you will see frequent references to stages and grades. In their writing and research about prostate cancer, the doctors organize their reports according to the stages and grades of the cancers they're studying. Their reports on prostate cancer survival rates, with treatment, are classified primarily by the stage and grade of the cancers. Most research and statistical reports are categorized that way. So, you need to know the grade and stage of your cancer if you want to know the odds that apply to you.

Typically, a urologist chatting with his peers might say, "This sixty-two-year-old fellow presented with a C tumor, Gleason 6. Otherwise seemed in good shape so I. . . ." What does that jargon mean? The "C" is the stage. The "Gleason 6" is the grade.

As we get into this critical subject it is time to define some other terms. When the docs say "screening," they mean surveying a number of apparently well men to see if any suspicion of prostate cancer exists.[1]

Screening is not the same as "diagnosis." Diagnosis is the individual examination of a patient to discover whether he has anything wrong with him and what that might be, and the further pursuit of detailed knowledge of his condition. Some of the diagnostic tests yield information for staging and grading. Specifically, these include the DRE (digital rectal exam), the PSA (prostatic specific antigen blood test), and the sonogram (the ultrasound pictures). Various scans of your body and studies of your cancer cells will contribute to classifying your cancer, as we will see.

Your doctor should tell you the stage and grade of your cancer, although these can change with time and further testing. What these tests yield is your *clinical* stage. If you have an operation, microscopic studies of the resulting tissues will yield a *pathological* stage. They could differ. Knowing your stage and grade will help you develop a realistic perspective and become an informed participant in your treatment.

I've come across two kinds of cancer patients in my studies. One will read everything about prostate cancer he can find. The other wants to know only what his doctor tells him and does not want to confuse himself with details that may not apply to his case.

If you are a person who wants to know about his disease in depth, remember to avoid the freshman Psychology 101 syndrome in which you find yourself suffering every phobia and neurosis in the textbook. Some of the professional literature can be blunt to the point of brutality.

For example, this is one of the introductory paragraphs repeated in each issue of the periodical publication *PDQ State of the Art* physician's information cancer treatment letter of the National Cancer Institute:

> Survival of the patient with prostatic carcinoma is related to the *extent of tumor dissemination.* When the *cancer is confined to the prostate* gland the disease is frequently curable; median survival in excess of five years can be anticipated. Patients with *locally advanced cancer* are not usually curable and a substantial fraction will eventually die from their tumor. Median survival of such patients however may be as long

as five years. If prostate cancer has *spread to distant organs,* it is not curable by current therapy. Median survival is usually one to three years and the majority of such patients will die from prostatic cancer. Even in this group of patients, however, indolent [meaning extended] clinical courses lasting for many years may be observed. (Emphasis mine)

These are either hopeful or grim tidings for the newly identified PCa victim, depending on his own cancer stage.

It is true that approximately one in four victims of the disease eventually will die of PCa but many of those will live out almost as many years as their age cohort in the nonafflicted population, some longer. Remember, half of the men who contract the disease are seventy years old or older at the time, and if you're seventy and in reasonably good health and have no disease, the insurance actuarial tables give you eleven years more of life. Depending on your age and the character—that is, the stage and grade— of your individual cancer you could match or exceed that despite the illness.

Age, overall health, and life expectancy are major factors in treatment decisions. Age is not applied to staging but is critical to your doctor's judgment. Donald Gleason, M.D., who developed the grading system, wrote in a National Cancer Institute monograph in 1988: "Other factors being equal, a group of older men will die sooner than a group of younger men. After age fifty, the changes per decade in the normal death rate are as great or greater than the changes related to tumor stage and grade."

The phrases I've emphasized in the NCI paragraph above, such as "extent of tumor dissemination," offer the key to the physician's mental exercises as he plans his assessment of his patient's condition and begins to think about treatment. He should leap to no conclusions about treatment until he is satisfied that the cancer is properly staged and that you, the patient, are sufficiently informed to participate in the treatment decision, at least to some degree.

This material grows somewhat technical, but it will undergird your understanding of what comes later.[2]

Staging Your Cancer

As an introduction to staging, think of prostate cancers as localized, regional, or distant. *Localized* means the tumor is confined to the prostate gland or within the capsule itself. *Regional* means it has spread to tissues just outside the capsule, perhaps to the seminal vesicles adjacent to the capsule just under the bladder. *Distant* means it has metastasized to places beyond the immediate vicinity, perhaps to lymph glands, bones, or other organs of the body.

Only three or four years ago, about a third of all cancers discovered were localized. The others had spread to some extent. With the advent of the PSA test, currently 50 to 75 percent of the newly discovered cancers are localized. This should mean for the future that thousands more men through early discovery will have a vastly improved chance for total cures. It will take several years for the mortality statistics to register this hopeful trend. Meanwhile, it is obvious that awareness and early discovery will be good for you.

For medical purposes, staging must be far more specific than these generalized definitions. Merely identifying a particular group by saying all men in it have a "localized" cancer is insufficient for the kind of comparisons and empirical guidance your doctor requires. Staging is not only an attempt to distinguish between apples and oranges but to identify what kind of apple and what kind of orange.

Any number of staging systems have been devised and there are frequent conferences, studies, and debates on standardizing staging. Researchers, especially, seek a uniform system that correlates with the clinical course of patients and assures students of the disease that they are using consistent and related definitions. Entire volumes report on meetings on this subject with doctors seemingly splitting infinite hairs trying to agree on precise definitions. To underscore the importance of precision, reports on treatments, experimental attempts at cures, and analyses of newly developed therapies invariably begin by describing the stages of patients' prostate cancers.

Your physician wants to know how many men with your precise stage and grade have been treated in a specific way and the successes and failures of that treatment before he subjects you to the procedure. The common base of such statistics relies on staging and grading accuracy.

Understanding staging is critical to discussion of treatments and research results and to the kind of comparisons—my cancer next to your cancer—that the PCa patient invariably talks about with his fellow victims. However, don't resign yourself to a "stage-based" fate. There are many variables.

Staging Details

For our purpose, I've adapted, merged, and re-edited the clinical and pathological descriptions of the several stages from American Cancer Society publications and American Urologic Association and National Cancer Institute materials. The most generally used staging definitions start with a relatively simple A through D system. I will run through this most commonly used system. For information on other frequently used systems and other details on staging, please see part 2 of this book. Don't puzzle over some of the terms at this point.

STAGING—SHORT VERSION:

A—confined to prostate; not feelable by the finger

B—confined to prostate; can be felt; may be on one or both sides

C—mostly confined to prostate but some extension to exterior of capsule, to margins, or to seminal vesicles

D—extended (metastasized) away from capsule to lymph nodes, soft tissue, or bone

Each of these stages has substages, such as B1, C2, etc. The following listings and charts explain the details of the stages for your information, if you want it now, or for your later reference. If you read any medical literature on prostate cancer, you'll need the details. ABCD is easy to remember. Substages, of course, refer to increased volume and spread of the tumor.

STAGE A: a clinically undetectable tumor confined to the prostate itself. It cannot be felt (nonpalpable) by the urologist's finger. Stage A tumors are usually found by examining tissues from prostate surgery, that is, transurethral resections (TURPs), open surgery for benign problems, or through a transrectal ultrasound procedure.

A1—tumor well differentiated, possibly in one location only, three or fewer foci (clusters of microscopic tumor cells) within the gland, less than 5 percent of gland, Gleason grade less than 6. (Gleason grades are explained more fully in the next chapter.)

A2—tumor poorly differentiated, more than three foci, more than five percent by volume of the prostate tissue removed, a Gleason grade of 7 to 10

STAGE B: a palpable tumor confined to the prostate gland

B0—PSA elevated, negative digital rectal exam, positive biopsy

B1—a single tumor nodule in one lobe of the prostate, confined to the gland, tumor 1.5 cm (0.6 inch) or less[3]

B2—more extensive involvement of one lobe, size greater than 1.5 cm

B3—extensive involvement of two lobes of the prostate

STAGE C: a tumor localized to the prostate area but extending through the outer layer of the capsule, perhaps into the seminal vesicles or through the margin

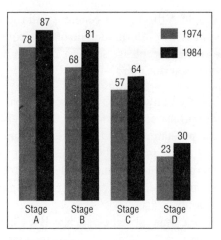

Fig. 1. Survival by cancer stage. This is a stage-specific chart of five-year prostate cancer survival rates (in percentages) for patients diagnosed in 1974 (a total of 20,166) in one study, compared with those diagnosed in 1984 (a total of 14,867). Five-year survival rates are up in every stage, and proportionally more so in stage B cancers. Remember that five-year survival figures for cases diagnosed in 1984 are from 1989. Source: American College of Surgeons Commission on Cancer patient care evaluation studies. Reprinted from *Ca—A Cancer Journal for Clinicians*, March/April 1993 (used with permission).

C1—extension through the prostate capsule or the seminal vesicles

C2—extension beyond the capsule perhaps involving the bladder outlet or obstructing the urethra, with larger volume of tumor than C1

STAGE D: this is metastatic disease, with tumors spread into areas "distant" from the prostate

D0—apparently localized disease but patient shows consistently elevated PSA or prostatic acid phosphatase level[4]

D1—tumor spread to local lymph nodes, in the pelvic area

D2—involvement of distant lymph nodes, metastases to bone or other organs

D3—D2 disease that has relapsed after endocrine (hormonal) treatment

The National Cancer Institute breaks out average survival times for each stage from the time of discovery of the cancer. It is encouraging to note that their percentages of five-year survival with treatment have an uptrend, possibly due to increasingly early discoveries through the PSA test and improvements in treatment procedures. For example, the current reports list for a stage A cancer a 90 percent chance of five-year survival. About two years ago, they listed only a 77 percent chance. The new figure for ten-year survival with a B1 cancer is 50 percent and with B2 cancers, 32 percent. The American Cancer Society reported in 1993 that with C and D stage tumors survival figures also have improved. So, we have a glimmer of hope that our chances of living longer with treatment seem to be improving in some categories. Indeed, the Cancer Society is even more encouraging. It says five-year survival rates for B stage cancers for those diagnosed in 1974 compared to 1984 show a survival rate increase of 13 percent—from 68 to 81. Some 1993 figures are even better.

Some experts in the field bemoan the fact that all the research and treatment improvement is not resulting in better survival. Nevertheless, afflicted men are living longer on average though they may not be completely cured.

Just How Sick Are You?

Understanding the PSA, Gleason Grades, and Such

Given your age and general health, the next question is how aggressive is your cancer and how fast might it grow?

ASSUME THEY'VE IDENTIFIED prostate cancer in you and started the imprecise task of staging and grading it. Recent improvements refined the process. It is not as specific or definitively prognostic as the docs would like, but they're getting closer.

Over the past three or four years, the prostatic specific antigen test (PSA) has become regarded as the most sensitive indication of cancer, more sensitive than the digital rectal exam (DRE), more sensitive than ultrasound.

Morton Schwartz, M.D., of the Memorial Sloan-Kettering Institute, once wrote that "PSA is the new marker of choice. In no other area of medicine has there been as dramatic an advance as this technique."

All three tests (PSA, digital rectal exam, and transrectal ultrasound) will be used, however, since, to quote Dr. Nash, "Nothing is 100 percent when dealing with prostate cancer. With an elevated PSA between 4 and 10, there's a 22 percent chance of cancer. (In this range, nonmalignant problems such as BPH could elevate the PSA.) If the PSA is more than 10, there's a 67 percent chance. But the PSA will miss somewhere between 17 and 30 percent of cancers and the DRE will miss more. With about 50 percent of the people I operate on, I can't even feel the cancer. They were found by PSA and transrectal ultrasound-guided biopsies or random biopsies."

Dr. William Catalona, widely recognized by his peers as a leading writer and researcher in prostatic affairs, notes that the majority of patients with a PSA greater than 10 ng/ml (nanograms per milliliter) will have some extension of their tumor. A nanogram is a millionth of a gram. In a more recent study, a PSA value greater than 20 ng/ml forecast cancer extension into the lymph nodes, yet only 40 percent of such patients turned out to have positive nodes.[1]

Until the late eighties, the DRE was the most relied upon diagnostic technique. Then the transrectal ultrasound (TRUS) became a confirmation of other findings. It is rarely a stand-alone cancer discovery method. Now the PSA ranks first. It is a test of the amount of a protein secreted exclusively by the epithelial cells of the prostate.

Drs. M. C. Wang, L. A. Valenzuela, and G. P. Murphy (formerly chief medical officer of the American Cancer Society) isolated the antigen in the late seventies. Application of the antigen as a "marker" for diagnoses was published in 1987 by Drs. Thomas A. Stamey and N. Yang and A. R. Hay. Advances in the use and measuring of PSA accelerated as its value became widely recognized.

Prostatic specific antigen is truly specific; no other organ of the body produces it. It is also gender specific: having no prostate, women cannot produce the antigen by themselves. Its concentration is increased in men with prostatic disease, including cancer. The detection of such small though significant parts testifies to the advances in laboratory measuring capabilities. Another advance is a urine PSA test and subsets of the test for BPH and cancer.

The final diagnosis is a three-legged stool. The PSA will miss some tumors. Some tumors will develop in areas of the prostate that the urologist cannot feel. And transrectal ultrasound (TRUS) will miss some. All three tests used in combination score a 97.5 percent discovery rate. Until the specificity of PSA was widely accepted, a prostatic acid phosphatase (PAP) assay, also a blood serum test, was a standard test for prostate cancer. An elevated PAP level is a strong indication of cancer, but it is affected by a variety of conditions and was found to yield many false positive readings. Its use in diagnosis is declining, but it is still used routinely as a clue to whether the cancer has spread out of the prostate and is about 70 percent reliable.

Your doctor's final staging judgment will await further tests and scans.

Medical journals or conference reports I read prior to 1992 insisted that PSA is not a staging tool. Principally, this is because a PSA of less than 10 ng/ml could indicate BPH or other noncancerous prostatic problems. Also sometimes a serious cancer may not yield a high PSA. Nevertheless, any PSA of 4 or greater is suspicious and that of 10 or more increases the possibility of a malignancy.[2]

More recently, however, continuing research into PSA shows it is useful in staging but still is not precise enough as a single determinant to stage disease in a particular patient. Dr. Joseph Oesterling of the Mayo Clinic, in Rochester, Minnesota, said that with the use of PSA in combination with the DRE and biopsy specimens, a "good estimate" of disease stage can be made. The PSA and the Gleason grade predict accurately whether a patient needs a pelvic lymph node examination to see if there is any tumor spread. Dr. Oesterling feels that PSA and Gleason grades at certain levels, which vary depending on the particulars of each case, can provide the physician with reliable guidance for his decision regarding surgical removal of the prostate.[3] Bone and CT scan results plus the findings of the probing finger also figure into the staging calculus.

As study of PSA continues, a new wrinkle is prostatic specific antigen density (PSAD). It is especially helpful in diagnosing men whose PSA falls into that indeterminate range of 4 to 10 where the reading could be BPH but may indicate cancer. There is more detail on this advance in chapter 26 in part 2.

No information about PSA is truly "old" since the test came into general use only in the late 1980s, but understanding of PSA values keeps improving. Several major studies now show a correlation between age and PSA. The reference to a range of 0 PSA to 4.0 ng/ml as indicating a normal prostate has been a general standard. A study conducted in six university centers led by thirteen doctors from around the country between May 1991 and September 1992 enrolled a total of 6,630 men fifty years old or older for a close study using PSA and DRE. Of 1,167 biopsies performed on the basis of suspicious findings, 264 cancers were found. PSA found more than DRE, but the combination of the two found more than either test alone, except for the eighty-plus age group.

The majority of cancers found in men under sixty-nine were organ-confined. This report cited a study that said five-year local tumor recurrence for this surgically treated group to be 2 percent and distant recurrence 1 percent. Older men showed a higher percentage of tumors that had been clinically understaged and PSA levels were correspondingly higher: 6.8 to 10.4 ng/ml compared with 6.3 to 9.0 ng/ml. In sum, the team reported:

> early detection programs yield a lower, yet still substantial, cancer detection rate in younger men, and there is a greater chance for detecting organ-confined disease in this age range. Younger men have the longest life expectancy and the most to gain from early cancer detection. Also, even though older men as a group have more advanced cancers and a shorter life expectancy, over half are candidates for curative therapy and may benefit from treatment if prostate

cancer deaths, the morbidity of metastases, or the unfavorable side effects of androgen deprivation therapy can be avoided.[4]

Dr. Oesterling said the normal (meaning very low likelihood of cancer) range of 0 to 4.0 ng/ml may be correct for men aged sixty, for younger men the range should be lower, and for older men, higher:

> for Caucasian men 40 to 49, normal range 0 to 2.5 ng/ml
> 50 to 59, 0 to 3.5 ng/ml
> 60 to 69, 0 to 4.5 ng/ml
> 70 to 79, 0 to 6.5 ng/mlx

So, for younger men a recognition of a lower range might discover more cancers. For older men, increasing the normal range might avoid needless ultrasound and biopsy procedures.[5]

Nevertheless, if your PSA is 4.0 or higher, most urologists now would want to biopsy you. The odds are worth the cost to you.

PSA also is a major marker for any progression of prostate cancer following treatment. Usually, the patient would have a PSA test at three, six, and twelve months following radiation and perhaps at two months and twelve months after surgery. The count comes down more slowly after radiation than after surgery. In either case, if after the count bottoms out it begins rising again there may be residual disease or recurrence.

A 1988 study emphasized the value of setting up a base-line PSA for an individual patient so that future PSA's could be better interpreted and any change noted. Thus, if the level of your PSA increases over time, further diagnostics can be intensified, perhaps to include biopsies; and following treatment, changes in PSA can be better used to estimate progression of disease, if any.

Note that PSA's may vary as much as 15 percent from day to day. Clearly, an annual exam, including a PSA, for men over forty is important. This study, edited by Dr. William Catalona and two Ph.D.'s, Donald S. Coffey and James T. Karr, raised some questions that have since been answered, such as "Is PSA a more reliable detection method for early prostate cancer than rectal exams or ultrasound?" Newer research proves it is, but it would be used in conjunction with the other methods, anyway, for thoroughness.

Or "What procedure should be followed for a patient who is found to have a 35 ng/ml level of PSA during a routine physical but who shows no other symptoms?" That one has not been answered fully, but Dr. Nash had a similar patient who showed negative on every test but the PSA, including three TRUS exams and biopsies. The doctor eventually withdrew prostatic tissue through the patient's penis, i.e., TURP, for analysis. Extensive cancer was discovered in the central zone of the prostate.

One report includes a story of a clinical scientist, no symptoms, who ran PSA tests on his own blood in the course of examining the potential value of setting up routine PSA testing at his own medical institution. The test found a PSA level of 28 ng/ml. A complete physical six months earlier had shown no prostate abnormality. The scientist had frozen samples of his own blood serum spanning ten years. These were thawed and assayed for PSA and PAP. The PAP was normal in all specimens. The PSA was stable and under 4 ng/ml for the first five years. Then a steady increase appeared. When the scientist saw this rising pattern of close to 5 ng/ml per year he sought an exam by a urologist who diagnosed a stage C prostate cancer. A course of radiation treatments followed.

This shows that a pattern of rising PSA values over time can be a powerful clinical tool, better than trying to compare a single PSA reading against some generally agreed-upon normal level.

The Gleason Grade

Clinical staging (the A–D or other staging system) must be augmented by histological grading for more accurate understanding of the life-threatening potential of the cancer and its eventual treatment. "Histological" has to do with the structure of the cancer cells themselves. The clinical stage, Dr. Gleason points out, deals with how far the cancer has progressed; the histological scale comes from microscopic examination of biopsy tissues.

The "Gleason scale" grades and seeks to predict the tumor's biologic malignancy. It expresses the risk of progression and the probability of death from the cancer. Microscopic examination of tumor cells obtained through biopsies reveal five major different but recurring cell patterns. From one to five of these patterns may be found in a specimen. The pathologist identifies the two predominant patterns on a scale of one to five, adds the scales of the two principal patterns together and obtains the final Gleason grade.[6] The grade is based on whether the cancer cells are clearly, individually defined ("differentiated") or irregular, not clearly separate and defined (not "differentiated"). So, $1 + 1 = 2$, the lowest and you might say "best" end of the scale; $5 + 5 = 10$, the highest end. Doctors classify a grade of 7 or above as indicative of future trouble, but that, too, depends on other factors. So in practice there are five "scales": the Gleason grade (histological), the stage (A–D), your age, your general health, and the genetic (DNA) makeup of the cancer cells themselves, generally referred to as "ploidy."

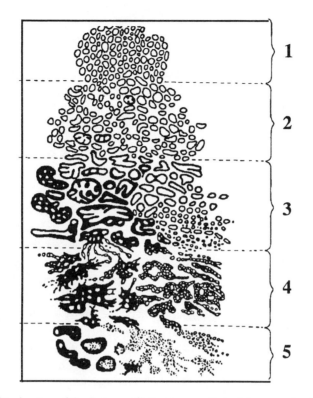

Fig. 2. This drawing of the various cell structures pathologists see under the microscope in a prostate cancer specimen is the guide for determining the Gleason grade of a
cancer. The top of the array (section 1) shows cells that are differentiated from each
other and yet are regular in their appearance. As we progress down the chart, we see
that the cells become more and more differentiated from each other and are increasingly irregular. When urologists speak of "differentiated," they are thinking of sections
1 and 2; "moderately differentiated" would be sections 2 blending into 3, and "poorly
differentiated" would be portions of section 3, and 4 and 5. The pathologist selects the
two most dominant patterns in the specimen and adds them together for the final
Gleason grade. For example, if 2 and 4 were dominant, the Gleason grade would be 6.
If the specimen were predominantly similar to section 4, the grade would be 4 plus 4, or
8. From D. F. Gleason, M.D., "Histologic Grading and Clinical Staging of Carcinoma
of the Prostate," in M. Tannenbaum, ed., *Urologic Pathology: The Prostate* (Philadelphia:
Lea and Febiger, 1977), pp. 171–197. Used with permission.

Remember that cancer cells are abnormal. They do not behave like the
normal cells in the body. Loosely speaking, they present their own DNA
patterns. They become independent of the rules of cell birth and death
that govern normal cells. It is the growth and independent spread of cancer
cells unregulated by normal cell guidelines that makes them dangerous.

During the last few years various studies have closely related the

Gleason grade with life expectancy: the more undifferentiated the cells, the more dangerous the tumor. Indeed, insurance companies may offer a policy to a prostate cancer survivor whose treatment appears to have been successful but will hesitate and perhaps refuse insurance if the Gleason tests show poorly differentiated cells, regardless of the clinical (A–D) stage assigned. Discussions of a patient's condition usually include whether his cancer is "differentiated" or "undifferentiated."

Ploidy, the News from Flow Cytometry about Your Cancer Cells

Flow cytometry (cell analysis) these days is an almost standard hi-tech examination of cells from biopsy or operating tissues. Development of lasers, computers, and advanced microscopes and techniques made cell study easier and more efficient. Flow cytometry analyzes one hundred to two hundred cells per second, whereas conventional microscopy may take several hours to analyze one hundred. It studies cell "ploidy" and other genetic factors in the cell for sharper definition of the cell's likely behavior.

In basic terms, "ploidy" characterizes the DNA within a cell, categorizing the different structures that may occur therein. DNA is the cell's principal building instructions, influencing its development, rate of growth, and ability to reproduce itself. Tumor cells may be classified as "diploid," "tetraploid," or "aneuploid." Things are complicated slightly by the fact that normal prostate cells are diploid, too. For our purposes it's enough to know that these terms indicate certain qualities of a cancer cell and its nucleus.

The different types are identified by the pattern refracted laser light produces on a cathode ray tube screen. The screen displays a grid. When the computer "reads" the refracted laser beam it projects a curved line, similar to a distorted bell curve. The three classes of ploidy each reflect a distinctive curved line pattern, as on a graph.

Flow cytometry uses both the refracted laser light and a DNA index of nonprostatic tissue as references. Properly used, this method is very sensitive. However, it is not specific enough to be a stand-alone diagnostic tool, because it depends on the quality of patient tissues, and for such a fine test, those tissues aren't uniformly gradable.

There's not total agreement on interpretations of ploidy. The different ploidies may relate to the age of a group of cells, and each ploidy type seems to have its own degree of aggressive growth or its ability to reproduce and rate of reproduction. An aneuploid reading is thought to be a sign of a more aggressive tumor. Several physicians told me they have never lost a patient to a diploid tumor that stayed diploid (the ploidy can change). Why ploidies differ and why some augur a more dangerous cancer than others is still hidden in the labs. Considerable research continues in this field, especially as to the higher threat to the patient of the aneuploid type.

Although the subject strains my meager knowledge of cellular biology, I'm fascinated by the discussions at medical meetings that speculate on the interactions of various types of cells and by the identification and duties of the assorted genes in our makeup. But one critic focused on reality when he rose at a medical conference I attended and said to the biologists, "This stuff is fascinating, but the double helix of DNA was discovered fifty years ago and you guys still haven't come up with anything specific we can do about bad cells."

Other Tests: Bone Scans, MRI, CT "Cat"

As we know from my experience, once your urologist suspects prostate cancer you'll endure several other tests. Some of these will play a role in staging, others produce medical information necessary to your treatment. The doctor may order an IVP, an IntraVenous Pyelogram, in which a medium, commonly called a dye[7] although it is not a dye, is inserted into your veins to better outline the kidneys and bladder and other organs. The IVP checks the condition of associated plumbing and organs, particularly of the bladder. It will find obstructions of the ureter, if any. It is not a cancer scan.

Your physician may order a bone scan, looking for bone abnormalities and any indication your cancer involves bone, and a CT "cat" scan (Computerized Tomography) to look for problems in lymph glands or soft tissues of the area for any extension of the tumor. The CT scan can be quite helpful. It can see into the interior of some organs. It may find unsuspected tumors of the kidneys, the pancreas, or other organs in addition to possible spread of the prostate cancer. As I mentioned, you've never had such a sharply focused peek at your insides before.

MRI, or magnetic resonance imaging, is being used more and more frequently as its technology improves and technicians gain more skill in reading its output. Both CT and MRI are used to evaluate pelvic lymph nodes, as well. We have many lymph nodes in our lower abdomen. The prostate drains into them and the lymph system processes the "waste." This is why metastases of prostate cancer frequently lodge first in the nodes.

MRI is not xray. It is a reflection of the passage of magnetic currents through the body and organs and so does not add to the buildup of xray radiation one accumulates in the course of various diagnostic procedures. New and smaller rectal probes for MRI have shown excellent resolution and thus the ability to pick up prostatic cancer, especially in lymph nodes or the seminal vesicles, although it may not spot any tumor smaller than half a cubic centimeter.[8]

A negative bone scan does not mean absolutely that no metastasis exists. Remember the "nothing is 100 percent" statement. The erring cells may be too small to be seen except microscopically. Nevertheless, a negative bone scan is good for the patient's morale and likely will result in a lower staging designation than otherwise. A positive bone scan and a high PSA, since the PSA is directly related to the volume of cancer present, is not good news; it will stage the patient as a D2 and thus make further elaborate staging unnecessary.

Lymph Node Dissection

Although ultrasound, MRI, and CT scans may be used to check lymph nodes, physicians also assess possible metastases through "surgical pelvic lymphadenectomies." This is removal of most of the lymph nodes draining the prostate. Checking the lymph glands can be a part of staging. It is routinely done preliminary to a retropubic (from the front) radical prostatectomy; and it may be done as a separate procedure before a perineal (through the crotch) radical prostatectomy.

One of urological surgery's controversies is whether to proceed with surgical removal of the prostate when lymph nodes show positive cancer. In the surgical procedure, tissue taken from the lymph nodes in the operating room is quick frozen and immediately analyzed in pathology. Only a few years ago, if that section were positive, surgical removal of the prostate was abandoned. That is no longer a universal attitude. Today many surgeons, including the Mayo group, continue with surgery even if the node contains a small amount of tumor.

Dr. Nash said, "If the node has only a small amount of tumor in it, I'll go ahead with the procedure and then I'll give hormonal blockade. I've only backed out of one surgical procedure in the past four or five years where the lymph node was that big (he held up his thumb and forefinger to show a size about that of a peanut) and we just backed out . . . didn't do the surgery."

Frequently, when lymph node invasion is suspected—perhaps by the appearance of an enlarged node in a MRI or CT scan—a fine needle will be inserted in the most suspicious area of the node, guided by the scan, and tissues withdrawn for biopsy. This is technically not a lymphadenectomy, just a biopsy.

An example of this procedure involved a former shipmate of mine, Jack Pennington, who happens to have a couple of doctors in his family and so went through the entire menu of tests, including this one. His prostate cancer was found at age sixty-nine. He is a long-distance runner and wins marathons in his age group. Jack tested with a normal PSA and his Gleason grade was in the midrange. Scans showed enlargement of the lymph nodes, raising suspicion of tumor extension. So Jack went through the process of having a needle stuck through his skin into the node. Despite the enlargement, the biopsy showed no cancer in the nodes, merely fibrous tissue, and the benign enlargement was blamed on his athletic activities.

Laparoscopic Pelvic Node Dissection

Metastases into the lymph nodes can be critical to staging your cancer. One of the major factors in understaging, which can lead to errors in treatment, is the enigma of the lymph nodes.

Laparoscopy for men who are to be irradiated was only rarely done when I was being examined and staged. So we didn't know, and I still don't, the status of my lymph nodes. My assorted scans seemed OK, no suspicions were raised, and the likelihood of any gross invasion of the lymph nodes is minute. I'd like to know, but unless my PSA rises or Cy Nash finds something to frown about I'll skip that drill.

MRI and CT scans frequently can detect whether the nodes are enlarged, but can't always peer into the interior of them. Laparoscopy is an advance in techniques. This is a method you've read about in operating for endometriosis, kidney problems or gallstones, hernia, appendicitis, cancer of the colon, or other abdominal problems. In laparoscopy, the abdominal cavity is inflated with CO_2. Instruments and a small camera are inserted through incisions far smaller than the typical surgical cut. The surgeon can see clearly in the area and, in prostate cancer matters, could excise lymph node tissues, withdrawing them through the incision.

Popular literature has described this process as "performing a hysterectomy through the belly button." It's not quite that easy. It is a full operation and takes about as much time as other abdominal surgery. However, trauma and aftereffects to the patient are minimized. Laparoscopy could make lymph node assessment feasible prior to radiation treatment. In a surgical removal of the prostate, a lymph node tissue sample is routine once the surgeon is "in there." Prior to radiotherapy, or the use of implanted radioactive seeds or cryosurgery, your doctor might do a laparoscopic removal and examination of the nodes. Knowing definitely that cancer is or is not in the lymph nodes would affect staging and treatment. This could become standard procedure on patients with moderately elevated PSAs, high Gleason grades, or palpable stage C disease.

Summary

All this probing and scanning and testing and lab work attempts to answer only a few critical questions: Is there a cancer present? If so, how much cancer is there? How aggressive is it? Has it spread beyond the prostate capsule and, if so, where? Given your age and general physical condition, what does it mean to your longevity? Do we do anything about it and if so, what?[9]

Now I have my stage, B2/C, and my grade, Gleason 6, and all my test results. I've also committed to the radiation route. The next step is the TURP.

8

Treatment Options
They Want YOU to Decide!

**It is inappropriate for the physician to prescribe
the right treatment. It is appropriate for the patient to choose it.**
DR. JOHN E. WENNBERG, Dartmouth Medical School, a leading researcher
into the consequences of prostate cancer therapies

THE QUESTION OF DECIDING on a treatment course now is complicated by medical reports, and recent press and TV coverage, on whether the prostate cancer patient should be treated at all. You may face this dilemma. So, I have a question for Dr. Wennberg and those colleagues who advocate the "watch and wait" theory.

Just how, doctor, is the untutored, under-read, medically ignorant patient, probably half traumatized from the shocking news of his affliction, supposed to select his own treatment? Here is a guy who barely knows a prostate from a kidney, moves his lips when he reads medical literature, and can't tell aspirin from Tylenol and you want him to write his own life-preserving Rx?

He can't. But he can participate, after advice and counsel from his urologist. Some urologists will expect more participation than others. We expect some sensitivity from a physician, so he should protect you from an utterly unsuitable therapy for your particular condition.

"Watch and wait" is termed "expectant management" by the doctors. Facing a smaller tumor in a man older than seventy-five, of limited life expectancy, Cy Nash might wait. Otherwise, he does not want to wait until the tumor grows and becomes incurable. He asks, "How are we going to make a dent in the 38,000-plus deaths a year if we don't treat early while the cancer may be curable?"

Dr. Wennberg was one of several researchers whose conclusions appeared in the May 26, 1993, issue of the *Journal of the American Medical Association.* They attempted to measure the effectiveness of various treatments against simply observing a patient and doing nothing, unless signs of troubles arose. They observed that the patient will suffer the procedures and consequences of any of the invasive therapies probably long before he would suffer the direct consequences of his cancer, given the slow-growing nature of most prostate cancer tumors.

They stated, "The patient will experience the impact of any complications sooner than he will experience any benefits of treatment: every patient who accepts invasive treatment faces some risk of complications, regardless of whether he eventually experiences the benefits of treatment.

The doctors are correct. The problem is if you wait until you know the tumor will hurt and possible kill you, it may be too late for treatment that intends to be curative. Except for men already in metastasis beyond curability, even prostate cancer therapies that intend to be curative are preventative, in the sense that they aim to keep the cancer from progressing. And the basic problem is that despite all the analyses available, no one can positively identify a dangerously aggressive tumor in its earlier and possibly curative phase.

"Tell me which tumors will progress and which won't," says Dr. Nash, "and I'll make the treatment decision easy for you. Even low volume, low Gleason grade, stage A, tumors can grow over time and cause death, although at lower rates than higher grades and stages.

"Most cancer therapy produces immediate side effects prior to the patient's realizing the hoped-for benefits, but we're trying to preserve life in the future."

Treatment Options

These are the treatment methods for prostate cancer:
—expectant management: waiting, watching, regular check-ups
—surgery, removal of prostate
—radiation, either external beam or implanted radioactive seeds
—freezing, circulating liquid nitrogen with probes to destroy tumor
    tissue
—hormonal treatment, androgen-suppressing drugs or orchiectomy
    (removal of testicles) or combinations, including antiandrogens
—chemicals, cytotoxic (aimed at killing cancer cells)
—combinations or series of the above
—assorted experimental therapies, used solely and in combination
    with traditional treatments; these include lasers, heating, and
    very early androgen blockade
There are other, strictly experimental, approaches. Biologists, delving deeply into genetics, the basic building blocks of our bodies, wonder if our own "suppressor genes" can be augmented and mobilized to prevent can-

cer cells from forming; or if we can find genes that will stop the process of metastasis by which "bad cells" travel in the body, take root in new sites, and develop their own destructive—to us—sources of nourishment.

Probably there are advocates of still other treatments, such as hypnosis or the chanting of incantations or dancing around in fright masks. I invested a great deal of time into trying to draw a grid of various stages and grades of prostate cancer with treatment options opposite each category— a sort of shorthand, charted overview of diagnoses and therapeutic choices. It became more complicated and confusing than simple prose. There are too many variables and too many possible consequences of treatment modes cum patient conditions. Better, I concluded, to broad-stroke the basics and leave the complex fine points to the doctors and their patients. It is a disease of discrete interpretation for each individual.

Certainly each of the direct treatment modes might be strengthened by positive mental attitudes, confidence in one's physicians, a sense of humor, and deliberate mind conditioning or control. I don't doubt that throwing myself into this book and challenging the cancer to give up its secrets has helped me so far. At least, the effort has taught me not to mull over things I can't help.

So, you and your doctor have a number of facts at hand. Do you go for treatment immediately or do you wait and see?

Here are some of the things you need to know (and you need to know them for the treatment decision, too):

—your age and general health, your life expectancy

—the stage of your cancer

—the Gleason grade of your cancer

—the "ploidy" of your tumor

—the experience of other men with similar readings (from reading and from your doctor)

—the effect on your mind and your behavior of knowing you are living with an untreated cancer inside you

—the downside of treatment relative to your quality of life, including treatment of possible side effects, possible permanent loss of potency, at least short-term pain and loss of recovery time (see assessments of other treatments herein)

—possibility of incontinence for a while or forever (small chance)

—possibility of death now (very small chance; less than 1 percent with surgery if you are under seventy-five) instead of several years in the future (depends on status of your tumor)

We will deal with "watching and waiting" in this chapter and each of the standard therapy options in chapters to follow. A more detailed examination of individual methods and their consequences is in part 2, so that if you want to focus on only one or two of them we'll spare you the details of the others.

Watching and Waiting

Until recently, only a minority of prominent physicians and medical educators advocated "expectant management," delaying treatment of localized cancers because they may never threaten their host or because a patient of relatively advanced years may die of something else before the cancer causes problems. If their assessment of the early tumor suggests it is not active they'll update their diagnosis on a regular basis but not treat unless some aggressive activity appears. Thus they hope to help the patient avoid costly and possibly risky treatment.

Lay opinions may have changed, or at least been thoroughly shaken, in May 1993 when the *Journal of the American Medical Association* (*JAMA*) published two related articles (and an editorial) comparing quality-of-life adjusted survival time for patients treated with radical prostatectomies or radiation and patients untreated but carefully followed.[1]

Two groups reported for the Prostate Patient Outcomes Research Team. Dr. Craig Fleming, of Oregon Health Sciences University, was lead author for a report analyzing expected outcomes of watchful waiting compared to radiation or surgical initial treatment for A and B tumors in men sixty to seventy-five years of age. Grace Lu-Yao, Ph.D., M.P.H., of Dartmouth Medical School, was lead author of an article based on a study of radical prostatectomies in a 20 percent sample of male Medicare beneficiaries aged sixty-five or older.

An accompanying supportive editorial, "Management of Clinically Localized Prostatic Cancer, An Unresolved Problem," was written by Dr. Willet F. Whitmore, Jr., of Memorial Sloan-Kettering Cancer Center, a longtime advocate of the watchful waiting approach.

Using a complex comparison formula, the Fleming report declared in most cases the potential benefits of therapy are small enough that the choice of therapy depends on the patient's preferences for various outcomes. In short, what they're saying is that in A and B tumors, accurately staged, treatment seems to make very little difference in the life expectancy and quality of life of many men and that watchful waiting is a "reasonable alternative to invasive treatment." In fact, a number of doctors, a minority, have been making this argument for years. The Fleming article adds statistical evidence to their position and does not speculate on the effects of improved treatment techniques across the years on the statistics included in its studies.

Fleming's group said further, "We could find no study or group of studies in the medical literature that definitively supports the benefits of either treatment [that is, radiation or surgery] over watchful waiting."

I caution again that the report is intensely detailed and its particulars highly qualified. The decision analysis is a complex process. The report noted a range of uncertainty about the risks and benefits of treatment but said,

> in patients with well differentiated tumor grades, based on clinical staging, treatment at best offers limited benefits in terms of quality-adjusted life expectancy and may result in harm to the patient. Among patients with moderately or poorly differentiated tumors, if we use the most optimistic assumptions about treatment efficacy, then patients aged 60 to 65 years would benefit from either radical prostatectomy or external beam radiation therapy, compared with watchful waiting.
>
> However, in most other cases, treatment offers less than a 1-year improvement in quality-adjusted life expectancy or decreases the quality-adjusted life expectancy compared with watchful waiting. Invasive treatment generally appears to be harmful for patients older than 70 years.

Lu-Yao and her team analyzed probabilities for men sixty-five or older. They considered sexually active men in average health for their age. In all, they studied 20 percent of all male Medicare beneficiaries in the fifty states and the District of Columbia, a total of 10,980 radical prostatectomies in the years 1984 through 1990. There were 5.75 times as many such operations performed in 1990 as in 1984. There were wide variations geographically. From 1988 to 1990, in the New England and mid-Atlantic states, rates for the operation were below 60 per 100,000 male Medicare beneficiaries: in the Pacific and Mountain regions, rates were equal to or above 130 per 100,000, more than twice as many, an inexplicable geographic difference.

When published in *JAMA*, these studies evoked front-page headlines throughout the country. The *Washington Post* proclaimed "Little Benefit Seen in Prostate Surgery." The typical press report did not make clear that one of the reports was limited to men sixty-five and older and the other to men sixty to seventy-five. About 12 percent of prostate cancers will be discovered in men younger than sixty. That's about 20,000 a year.

One of the members of the Fleming report team, Dr. John Wasson of Dartmouth Medical School, said in a press conference, "We're doing a lot in this country, yet it is unclear that we know what we are doing."

Any urologist will concede that they cannot yet identify which tumors will progress and which won't, but we can assume thousands of urologists took substantial umbrage at being told they don't know what they're doing. They are removing tumors because in properly staged patients they can't take the chance the tumors will progress.

Before we base our treatment decision on these reports we should recognize that they contain some necessary assumptions. One is that the effect of a radical prostatectomy and of external beam radiation are equal, which, depending on the stage and grade of your cancer, may not be true. Another is that during the time a tumor takes to metastasize, a certain number of men over sixty-five will die of other causes. It assumes a number of survivors with prostate cancer will receive palliative treatment for metastases and while those symptoms are being controlled, an additional number of men will die of other causes. So, depending on the state of your cancer when it is discovered, the "no treatment" modality offers a sort of race between whatever else is out there after you and your cancer's progression.

But there are other factors to consider. The Fleming study estimated treatment efficiency—either surgery or radiation—at 100 percent for well-differentiated tumors; 72 percent for moderately differentiated tumors; and 35 percent for poorly differentiated tumors. Whether both modes offer equal results is highly debatable. Many doctors don't think anymore they are that equal.

Longevity comparisons of treatment versus no treatment, based on high treatment efficiency, gave a difference in outcomes of less than 0.1 years for all age groups, barely more than one month. For patients younger than seventy, treatment provides some marginal benefit, according to the study. Using the highest estimates of treatment efficiency, younger men with high-grade tumors survived 3.5 years longer with treatment than without. In most cases, however, treatment yielded less than one additional year of quality-of-life adjusted survival. Using lower estimates of treatment efficacy, watchful waiting yielded equal or better outcomes for men of average health.

These studies tend to reinforce the position of Dr. Willet F. Whitmore, Jr., of the Memorial Sloan-Kettering Cancer Center in New York. Although Dr. Whitmore is now essentially retired he was one of the most highly regarded doctors in his field and almost an icon at Sloan-Kettering. In February 1991, Dr. Whitmore and associates noted that data is relatively limited on the natural evolution of localized cancers. In other words, "What happens if you leave them alone?"

They reviewed the histories of seventy-five patients with clinical stage

B1, B2, and B3 prostatic cancers. Forty-six ultimately had treatment; some with iodine-125 implantation, some with TURPs, and some with hormonal therapy. These men had no treatment for the first year after diagnosis, a procedure to which they agreed after discussions with their physicians.

After 20 or more years of following these patients they found little difference in the survival of those treated—at some stage in the cancer's progression—and those that did not progress and were untreated. For example, of six B2 patients followed 15 to 20 years, one was alive, the report says, without therapy 186 months (15.5 years) after diagnosis with local progression only; three were alive after interval therapy. Two with local and distant progression died with metastases at 16.5 years and 19 years respectively; these had received hormonal therapy at 7.25 years and 8.5 years respectively, and were in clinical remission at the time of death.

Dr. Whitmore's point is that it is important to assess the potential evolution of a tumor and perhaps avoid curative therapy. But at no point does he assert that his team in their research found the key to that assessment.

The B2 patients did the most poorly, but even of those, more than half survived ten years and 25 percent eighteen years. Some had interval treatment. The trouble with this study is that any suffering or debilitation the patients might have endured is unreported. Some of us may not be interested in twenty years' survival, as a case in point, if the last two are in severe pain and paralysis. However, the more recent reports do factor "quality of life" into their survival figures.

Maybe an incidental or a small tumor will never threaten its host's life. Maybe a significant percentage of treatments is unnecessary. Certainly treatment will depend on an individual patient's diagnosis and dynamics. The fact remains that physicians across the world are treating A1 and A2 cancers, as well as B1's, B2's, and B3's, routinely, except for A1's in older men.

As recently as 1991, Dr. Deborah Markiewicz, University of Pennsylvania Hospital, and Dr. Gerald E. Hanks, Fox Chase Cancer Center, Philadelphia,[2] concluded in an exhaustive analysis of existing studies that A1 patients with moderate differentiation showed significant rates of symptomatic progression and that A2 patients, by definition with diffuse disease or poor differentiation, require definitive treatment. They noted that patients selected for observation only require careful follow-up for fifteen years, with physical exams, digital exams and consistent review of pathology, suggesting periodic biopsies.

Dr. Whitmore kindly sent me the script of his talk at a 1992 San Francisco National Conference. He continues to make a case for studying patients with stage A and B cancers in whom possible curative therapy may be unnecessary. Close observation and improved diagnostic procedures would permit effective action if that becomes required, he says. Patients with low grade A and B lesions have a reasonably good outlook with or without treatment. Dr. Whitmore points out that survival rates between patients treated aggressively (radiotherapy or radical prostatectomies) and those managed expectantly (deferred treatment) indicate that freedom from cancer is not demanded for ten-year survival. He said,

> This, coupled with competing mortality (from other causes of death in older men) makes cancer cure a less compelling goal in prostatic cancer management. In contrast to clinically localized lung or pancreatic cancer wherein failure to "cure" usually means death from the disease within two years, the probability of survival at ten and even fifteen years appears remarkably similar with or without prostatic cancer cure. This fact does not challenge the worthiness of cancer cure as an ultimate goal but it does raise practical questions regarding the circumstances in which this goal need be pursued in the individual patient.

This is a critically important debate to prostate cancer patients. Already it appears to be affecting the judgments of men who genuinely need treatment. A Nash patient diagnosed with a B2 tumor and a high Gleason grade canceled a scheduled operation on the strength of the medical journal reports.

Some earlier "watch and wait" arguments relied heavily on Swedish studies. These raise some strong doubts. In socialized medicine countries, how much do treatment decisions depend on costs? Half the men in the studies had grade 1 cancers, raising doubt as to how many really had cancer in the first place. Follow-up periods were relatively short.

In an attempt to define more specifically the application of "conservative management" in localized cancers, a team of eleven researchers led by Gerald W. Chodak, M.D., University of Chicago Hospitals, examined 828 case records from six studies published since 1985. Their findings were reported in the *New England Journal of Medicine,* 27 January 1994, by Dr. Chodak and the team. Swedish and Israeli studies were included. Dr. Chodak is a professor of surgery and director of the Prostate and Urology Center at Weiss Memorial Hospital.

Dr. Chodak noted that because there is "no clearly superior therapy, marked differences in treatment recommendations [exist] in different regions of the United States and in Europe." Two other problems, reiterated in the study, are that (1) reliable methods of identifying life-threatening tumors early on aren't available and (2) critics find reasons to question the validity of various studies.

The report classified three grades of tumor: grade 1, Gleason sums of two to four; grade 2, Gleason sums of five through seven; grade 3, Gleason sums of eight through ten.

Mortality from prostate cancer among men with grade 1 or grade 2 tumors was 13 percent at ten years but was 66 percent among men with grade 3 disease. The report said, "Metastatic disease developed significantly more often with increasing tumor grade. By ten years after diagnosis, metastases had occurred in 19 percent, 42 percent, and 74 percent of men with grades 1, 2 and 3 respectively. The results clearly demonstrate that prostate cancer is a progressive disease when managed conservatively."

Differences between aggressive therapy (surgery or radiation) and "watchful waiting" at ten years are difficult to determine, the report summarizes, because treatment data based on tumor grade are lacking. With grade 1 or 2 the differences may be slight, especially since treatment may affect quality of life. The report made no judgment on grade 3 patients. It said that essentially the same outcome (as with aggressive treatment) can be achieved for at least ten years with initially conservative management of grades 1 or 2 cancers.

Thus for men with a life expectancy of ten years or less, "watchful waiting" was deemed a reasonable option. For men with a longer life expectancy, "watchful waiting" means a higher probability of living with metastasis and of dying from prostate cancer than if aggressive therapy is applied. The report called for new "management strategies for grade 3 cancers because neither surgery nor radiation substantially lowers the high rates of metastasis and mortality when these patients are treated conservatively."

This report will be influential in treatment decisions for grades 1 and 2 cancers, especially concerning older men. But the decision is turned back to us, the patients, making it more and more essential that we be as informed as is possible for a layman as we discuss our treatment with our physicians, who may or may not endorse aggressive treatments. The Chodak study says as much: "Whether a higher ten year disease-specific and metastasis-free survival for grade 1 or 2 cancer is worth the risk of complications associated with irradiation or surgery *should ultimately be the patient's decision.*" (Emphasis mine.)

As the treatment versus no-treatment debate continues, more specific research focuses on trying to find criteria for the decision. A persuasive report on the probable need for treatment of certain nonpalpable (the finger can't feel them) cancers joined the fray in the February 2, 1994, issue of the *Journal of the American Medical Association.* Dr. Jonathan I. Epstein and three colleagues of the Johns Hopkins departments of pathology and urology authored an article entitled "Pathological and Clinical Findings to Predict Tumor Extent of Nonpalpable (Stage T1c) Prostate Cancers."

A T1c cancer by definition is nonpalpable and is identified by a needle biopsy taken because of an elevated PSA. (It would be staged B0 on the A–D scale.) The team found that 84 percent of cancers clinically identified as T1c are significant and, if they had been palpable would have been classified for treatment. Of these only 51 percent were confined to the capsule and 34 percent showed extracapsular extension. They concluded that "most stage T1c tumors are moderate or advanced and many may become incurable before they become palpable."

The model they found most predictive of significant tumor was one that assessed PSA density (PSAD) at greater than 0.1 ng/ml per gram or that showed adverse pathology in needle biopsy samples. PSA density is a function of the PSA relative to prostate weight. I add again that I am over-simplifying their definition as the point here is not to teach us diagnostic arts but to argue that specifics may refute at least some aspects of the "no treatment" decision. In any event, simply because a tumor cannot be felt doesn't mean it lacks dangerous potential and none can be dismissed without going through the entire routine of tests and measurements. Needle biopsies can miss critical sites of tumor and some aggressive tumors will not elevate PSA tests proportionately to their potential virulence.

This debate will continue. It is basic, bringing into contention the gamut of prostate cancer detection efforts, including general screening, because if we are not going to treat early cancers why should we go to so much trouble looking for them? Thus into the fray comes Marc B. Garnick, M.D., of the Dana-Farber Cancer Institute of the Harvard Medical School. He wrote in *Scientific American,* April 1994, "If treatment is undesirable, it follows that screening asymptomatic men for evidence of prostate cancer is unnecessary and wasteful."

In a well-balanced article, Dr. Garnick noted the "no treatment" arguments in the Swedish study and the Fleming study and referred to the Chodak report, as well. But though he termed the studies "provocative," he found them "seriously flawed and thus far from definitive." Not all patients in the Swedish group, he points out, were selected randomly. Some were chosen because they had well-differentiated tumors and a disproportionate number were elderly or had other life-threatening disorders. Similarly, the Chicago study contained mainly elderly subjects. Dr.

Garnick commented that this imbalance put into question the studies' applicability to younger men. He continued:

> The conclusions of the Fleming group are problematic as well. At least some of the patients who were identified as having been followed with watchful waiting did not, in fact, go without treatment. They were given hormonal therapy early in the course of their disease. . . . Moreover, only sexually active men were selected: for them, impotence would reduce quality of life more than it would for other men. Hence [this focus] probably biased the findings against treatment.
>
> Thus, the benefits attributed to watchful waiting by (the Fleming group) may be smaller than has been claimed. In fact, uncritical interpretation of the findings reported in this and related studies may be leading many men who need treatment to opt for watchful waiting and to thereby lose their chance for a cure.

Just how serious are the risks? We'll get to that.

Dr. Nash examines the "watchful waiting" issue: "Why are so many prostate cancers understaged, some 50 percent of the cases we operate on? Because we got them tardily. Because PCa is a multifocal disease. It may not just be in one spot. It hides. In a rectal exam, there are multiple areas you can't feel. I'd say half the cases are multifocal and not in one area. That's why if you biopsy one area and the cells are well differentiated, another area could be totally undifferentiated. So, what you get in tests may not be what's there.

"Whether early (very small) cancer should be treated in all men is the question. Early cancer in older men may not mean anything, but early cancer in a man who may live another twenty or thirty years is very, very important. Give me an eighty-five-year-old man with a low Gleason grade and a negative bone and CT scan and I'll just see him every four months. If his PSA stays the same, we won't treat him. But the younger patient with the same lesion, we'll treat. He may have ten to twenty years for that thing to grow. If untreated, that person by age seventy may have metastases in his bones."

Dr. Nash shares with many of his colleagues skepticism regarding the "watch and wait" philosophies of the Patient Outcomes Team reports. He notes that "all cancer therapies produce side effects prior to the realized benefits of the therapy. The long-range goal is to prevent debilitation and death."

He suspects the formula used to assess quality of life and other factors in the studies was so complex it could be weighted toward the outcome desired. The studies reported in *JAMA* were funded by the U.S. Agency for Health Care Policy and Research, Rockville, Md., a government agency. This agency has sponsored many research projects including one several years ago that concluded that men who have had TURPs for BPH were threatened with shorter life spans.

This implied to urologists that perhaps these men were higher-risk patients at the initiation of treatment compared to men who had open benign prostatic surgery for their BPH. But the agency made no such distinction and, in effect, fixed on the TURP procedure and not on the condition of the patients.

Dr. Patrick C. Walsh of Johns Hopkins in the July 1994 *Journal of Urology*'s Urological Survey (pp. 255–256) strongly criticized Chodak-led reports in *New England Journal of Medicine* advocating expectant management. Writing as senior editor for a commitee of fifteen urologists, he noted the background section of the *NEJM* studies criticized previous studies of conservative management as "uncontrolled and unrandomized," and he asked, "How is this study any different?" He charged the studies with selection bias because the Whitmire, Johnsson, and Moskovitz reports excluded appreciable numbers of their patients. He noted also that 60 percent of the patients in the Chodak et al. report had grade 1 tumors and pointed out that at Johns Hopkins only 11 percent of patients undergoing radical prostatectomy have grade 1 disease. He conceded that the study authors had said that watchful waiting was reasonable for men with grade 1 and grade 2 tumors if their life expectancy is ten years or less but he remarked that this conclusion was "buried in the paper."

A layman might speculate that the growing sense of acrimony in this debate arises as doctors hear more questions and increased indecision from their patients. Or perhaps there are those among us who don't want to ask—or know—if our life expectancy is ten years or less.

Dr. Nash criticizes the Fleming and related studies because they include groups of Swedish low grade and stage prostate cancer patients, many of whom may not have had cancer at all. Half of these patients were diagnosed by aspiration biopsies (fluid rather than tissues withdrawn from the prostate), which are not considered totally reliable. The reports compared this group to a group of younger patients with more advanced and higher grade disease who underwent surgery.

Many of his colleagues, Dr. Nash believes, suspect built-in biases in government-sponsored studies tending toward more economic procedures. "Watch and wait" certainly is less expensive than therapy, especially in the short run, and economical medicine may particularly influence study outcomes in socialized medicine countries.

Dr. Nash concludes: "Tell me who to watch. I don't want to be the doctor the patient comes to later and says, 'Why didn't you treat me? Look at me now.' There was a doctor at one of the big clinics—this was before the PSA tests—who watched. A certain percentage of his patients died of prostate cancer. If he watched one hundred men and five of them died because he didn't realize their cancers were growing or spreading, I wouldn't want him to take care of me of I were one of the five.

"If you wait, maybe it will take four years to show progression, maybe eight years, and maybe never. But the tests are too uncertain. I rarely wait. The risks of the treatment procedures at that stage are very small. The risks of waiting are much higher.

"Of course, there are risks of consequences. But if we increase life expectancy, what if a small percentage of patients must use a pad or a napkin? They are living longer."

Dr. Whitmore's editorial concerning the May 26, 1993, *JAMA* reports said, "although any benefits of aggressive treatment over watchful waiting in terms of quality-adjusted life expectancy are often small in absolute terms, whether they should be considered negligible may be a decision best left to the individual patient."

He noted in a July 1993 article in *Cancer* that data used in "watch and wait" commentaries are "in many respects imprecise and inadequate," but that they are the same data on which current opinions regarding treatment methods are based.[3]

Whitmore and his co-authors concluded their report:

> We did not attempt to examine these important considerations (quality of life, possible side effects of treatment) . . . our analysis has attempted a global assessment of the consequences of three different therapeutic strategies on selected endpoints in up to 10 years of follow up of patients with apparently similar prostate cancers.
>
> Although it is evident that cure may be neither a necessary nor a rational objective for all patients with a clinically localized prostate cancer, the problem remains to predict accurately the need for and consequences of a particular management in an individual patient.

Your decision? Proper medical counseling must contribute to the decision. The physician recommends and must assist the decision by informing the patient of his options. "People are grasping for easy solutions," says Dr. Nash, "but must not be misled. Waiting means less chance of curing."

9

The Ray Gun or the Knife
You're the Prize in This Ongoing Debate

The game remains urologist-surgeons versus radiological oncologists and therapists, but the debate breaks down to what the individual patient needs—and wants.

DIFFERENT PEOPLE, DIFFERENT CANCERS, equal different treatments. Prostate cancer is a complex problem and so is determining the most suitable therapy. I have two professional magazines that devoted entire editions to prostate cancer treatments. Each has at least three times as many words as this book.

Addressing the issue of treatments, the medical world tries to set up some categories: (I know I've reported this earlier but why should you have to look it up?)

—localized, meaning A and B cancers primarily, those thought to be confined to the prostate

—advanced, including C's, and those with some extension, perhaps into tissues adjacent to or very near the prostate

—extension of cancer into the lymph nodes or metastasized elsewhere, or D's

—recurring or residual cancer (failure of primary treatment)

There's a treatment range for each. But the therapies do not necessarily fall into a proscribed category for every patient with a given stage and grade. This report does not intend to enable you to prescribe your own treatment. Its purpose is to help you enter into treatment discussions with your physician and to recognize the range available to you if you and your "team" decide therapy is desirable.

Your age, general health, and life expectancy, plus your clinical stage and grade, the other factors listed earlier, and your own hopes, fears, sense of destiny, and mental attitude will guide your decision. Your doctor will help interpret the medical clues: he will want you to assess the personal and psychological ones.

If you have an A1 cancer that appears to have a single location, a fairly low PSA, well differentiated, you may opt for conservative treatment, that is, careful watching and waiting, depending on your age (life expectancy). In the small number of studies tracking such patients for four years only a small percentage (in one study,[1] only 2 percent) progressed. In another, after eight years, 16 percent. Other studies are approximately in this range.

An A1 cancer may be indolent—just sit there—for years and even the pathologist's analysis of its virulence (Gleason grade and ploidy), while probably the best clue to any future activity, may not be predictive. Some patients, a relatively small number, have progressed and died when early treatment might have prevented advancement of the disease. Drs. Markiewicz and Hanks wrote that A1 patients with moderate differentiation "demonstrated significant rates of symptomatic progression . . . definitive treatment is warranted."

An A2 cancer (remember, the doctor's finger can't feel A's) is more likely to progress. Infrequently, also, an A2 will be discovered at surgery, when tissues can be closely analyzed, to have been understaged and will turn out to be a stage C or D disease. Various small studies showed excellent results from both surgical and radiological treatment, about 85 percent survival at five years and 67 percent at ten years. None of the patients was under sixty years of age at discovery. These figures compare with "age-matched men in the general population," in medical report vernacular.

In untreated A2 cancers, however, local progression in up to one-third of those in a study and 22 percent cancer deaths were reported.

Several articles I read presented tables showing patients' ages, stage and grade of cancers, and years of survival after treatment. You can look these up. Your doctor knows them. But I want to hedge on those and so may he. Obviously, it takes five years and ten years to accumulate five- and ten-year survival rates, so I tend to be a little dubious about stale statistics.

To go back to the mid-eighties for a start date may be misleading. Both surgical and radiation techniques and procedures have changed so much since then, we might look on the "old" statistics for trends but be inclined not to take them too precisely for today's decisions. The same mild skepticism applies to figures on negative consequences of surgery or radiation.

Most researchers have concluded that A2 cancers (more than 5 percent of the prostate involved) will suffer progression if left untreated.

Stage B cancers can be felt by the probing finger. The other diagnostic techniques signal the size of the tumor, and pathology can assess the possible aggressiveness. B's indicate the tumor has been there a while and survival rates with treatment for five-, ten-, and fifteen-year periods are slightly below those for A's. Clinically staged B2's turn out about 50 percent of the time to be C or even D cancers at surgery, when the pathological stage can be determined.

With the improvements in surgical techniques, the weight of medical opinion now seems to favor a radical prostatectomy when the cancer is confined to the prostate and the patient has a 10-year life expectancy. This would include A and B staged cancers. Some research leaders advocate radical prostatectomies for stage C, as well, plus other treatment.

With A and B tumors, and no lymph node invasion by the cancer, Dr. Stephen N. Rous (in his *Prostate Book*) favors surgery over radiation, based on his experience and on his concerns about the side effects of radiation. "X-ray therapy is clearly a second choice alternative to total removal of the prostate and should be first choice only for those who refuse surgery or whose health won't permit it."

He concedes that radiation therapy has produced very good long-term results in some patients. But many of these are alive with the prostate cancer still present, as documented by the high percentage of radiation patients who still have positive biopsies months and even years after treatment.

Now we've joined the argument that occupies a lot of research time and urologist versus radiologist debates. If your doctor thinks you fall into the category of "localized" cancer patients, he may say, "Look. You can have radiation or you can have this cancer surgically removed. You have to take part in this decision." Then he'll tell you the differences in the treatments, the possible outcomes and side effects, and the approximate costs of each. Legally, the doctor is required to explain your options.

He knows the risks of each procedure. He wants you to share the responsibility for possible impotence, incontinence, strictures, damage to the bladder or rectum, and possible recurrence of the cancer itself. With radiation, there's a 50 percent chance of some recurrence, and though some cells that resisted or were immune to the ray gun grow back very slowly, if at all, some will be serious and it is difficult to tell in advance in an individual patient. If you decide on surgery, the operation will include a pathological examination of your lymph nodes. If cancer is found, it means you have been understaged and will be reclassified with a stage D cancer. Unless a gross amount of cancer is found, some surgeons today will proceed with the operation and plan further postoperative treatment. (See chap. 16 on advanced cancer treatments.)

If you opt for radiation treatment and your various exams and tests raise your doctor's suspicions, he may want to examine your lymph nodes before you are zapped. The decision may depend on your PSA and Gleason scores. This can be done laparoscopically or, less precisely, with needle drawn tissues for biopsy if CT scans show enlarged nodes.

Even with a good report on your lymph nodes, if you are having surgery there's a chance your cancer may have been understaged and that some cells, perhaps microscopic ones, will remain in tissues that are not removed with the prostate itself. If that is the case, or is suspected, you may receive postoperative radiation treatments or hormonal blockade, or both. (See chap. 14 on surgery.)

Each procedure has its advocates and each its reports in medical literature showing percentages of recurrences after treatment, survival times, survival after recurrence, if any. Not all the studies are uniform, that is, they can't be compared to each other. There's also the matter of time and the fact that procedures and techniques continue to improve in each method, even though the basics haven't changed. Moreover, statistics on the seriousness of recurrence after radiation are difficult to come by. A climbing PSA or a suspicious DRE, or both, will lead to a repeat of the tests you remember so well. But even with a positive biopsy, interpretation isn't easy. Maybe the cancer is alive but stunned; maybe it is present but unable to reproduce. Lots of prostate brothers are walking around with posttreatment positive biopsies that are a decade or more old.

Indeed, there have been several reports, well researched, that equate radiation and surgery in terms of disease-free survival and long-term survival. But the arguments are not settled by any means, and urological surgeons are convinced that taking out the prostate altogether is a surer cure, perhaps preserving potency at least as frequently as radiation, which costs about 50 percent of patients their sexual prowess (and that percentage increases gradually over time). Note also that improvements in both procedures haven't been practiced long enough to allow absolutely reliable figures to emerge.

If you memorized this book so far, however, you know that Cy Nash believes only fifteen-year disease-free survival figures are meaningful and that any recurrence is a negative, as remaining cancer cells may grow and may change to more threatening ploidy status. It is also true that surgical patients have been selected for age and general health conditions so that broadly observed many were better risks to start with than were radiation patients. Moreover, in any study reaching back fifteen years, very few stage C patients received surgical therapy. That, too, is changing.

Dr. Charles B. Brendler, then of Johns Hopkins and now at the University of Chicago, stated emphatically to a postgraduate seminar in 1991 that "I believe there is increasing evidence to suggest that radiation therapy is not nearly as effective as was previously believed."

He discounted comparative studies, saying differences in staging procedures and study methods destroy their integrity. He also negated the argument that positive biopsies following radiation are inconsequential and that remaining cancer cells have been rendered biologically inactive, and he asserts that it is now known that a cancer that exists a year after radiation poses a greater risk of metastatic disease and death from cancer.

Dr. Brendler said that while it is impossible to draw meaningful conclusions from comparisons of overall survival rates (although that's an important figure to the patient) four items of evidence "strongly suggest" that radical prostatectomy is superior to radiation therapy in treating localized prostate cancer. He lists the four: disease-specific actuarial survival rates, comparative trials, local recurrence rates, and posttreatment PSA levels.

He cites a number of studies of recurrence of cancer even though he says the various studies are difficult to compare. In them, however, recurrences were fewer and took longer to appear with radical prostatectomies than with radiation as initial treatment. He reported data from a Stanford study of ultrasound-guided biopsies in eighteen men who had been treated by radiation more than eighteen months previously. Biopsies were positive for sixteen of the eighteen, and he concludes that many if "not most patients treated with radiotherapy will have residual prostatic cancer, and such men have an increased risk of recurrence."

The Stanford group performed biopsies on twenty-seven men who had had radiation therapy eighteen months earlier and ten out of the twelve who showed PSA levels less than 10 ng/ml had positive biopsies; all fifteen with PSA levels greater than 10 ng/ml also had positive biopsies.

He concludes, "There is now strong evidence that radical prostatectomy is superior to radiation therapy . . . furthermore the risks of urinary incontinence and impotence associated with radical prostatectomy have decreased dramatically in the past decade . . . therefore radical prostatectomy should be the treatment of choice for healthy men under seventy with localized disease." Here again, the diagnostic question arises: is it truly localized?

In a most emphatic statement, Dr. Thomas A. Stamey, chief of urology at Stanford Medical Center, wrote, "I have ceased using radiation therapy as a primary treatment for prostate cancer except for metastatic bone pain." He reached this conclusion after a study showing that 7,000 rads (as high as they go with the radiation beam) used as primary therapy cures only 20 percent of the patients and that at five years, the remaining 80 percent "have ominously high rates of rise in their PSA, suggesting clonogenic selection of more aggressive radiation resistant cells."[2]

Dr. Brendler's difficulty in finding precisely comparable reports is further confirmation that studies of patients whose treatments started in the seventies and even early eighties are yesterday's apples compared to today's oranges. The Walsh innovations in surgery date back only to 1982, so there are not many ten-year-old statistics related to those advances. Similarly, technical advances and improved skills in radiation therapy clearly separate today's probable long-term results from treatments of ten and fifteen years ago. Moreover, there are new variations on the external beam theme that improve focusing and intensity, including improved treatment planning through CT scans.

Implanted radioactive "seeds" offer another choice for consideration. New methods of implantation seem to be improving results but more time must pass before meaningful comparisons can be made with either surgery or external beam radiation treatment. Major advantages of implants include a very short hospital stay, a significant improvement in retention of potency, and avoidance of several of the possible side effects of other therapies. Younger men with localized cancers should inquire carefully of the possibility of this treatment.

So, make sure, as Cy Nash advises, that your own urologist is current in his reading, that he's attended recent conferences on trends and research in prostate cancer and can talk to you candidly about treatment choices, without a specialist's built-in biases. A National Cancer Institute conference recommended that physicians have information up to date and available to their patients, so make sure you ask both your urologist and, if appropriate, your possible oncological radiologist the proper questions:

—what is the probability of cure, mortality, complications, and other side effects of radical prostatectomy and radiation therapy?

—what are the risks of impotence and incontinence, partial or total, for either treatment?

—what may be, for me, the psychological consequences of either choice?

—what are the chances that the pretreatment tests and staging assessments may be off the mark, and what happens if they are?

—what are the comparative costs of the two treatment methods?

—at my age, whatever it may be, what are the threats to my quality of life and what are my chances of dying of prostate cancer before something else gets to me?

—say, for the sake of educating me, that whichever method we choose, my cancer recurs. Which initial procedure is most likely to avoid recurrence and which offers the best chance for a cor-

rective second (salvage) attempt? (The answer will depend
greatly on the staging of your cancer, but it is a good question to
ask your doctors to encourage them to tell you the total story. To
a man under seventy in good health most urologists would answer, "Surgery.")

The Turrible TURP
What It's Like to Go through the Operation

Now they've quit preaching and gone to meddlin'.
Old Mountain Anecdote, Anonymous

OK. WE'VE NOTED THE ELEMENTS of the treatment decision. Let's get to the treatment itself.

Three and a half hours from Gainesville, we tied down the Bonanza securely at Opa-locka airport, Miami, knowing there'd be no wild blue yonder available for several weeks. My pleasurable concentration on flying faded and my mind turned to that sneaky gland and my upcoming Trans-Urethral Resection. After all, it isn't one of those exotic operations, I told myself, if 350,000 men in the U.S. go through it every year.[1] As events turned out, Cy Nash would have to fill me in on the details afterward because I was out cold during the operation, unlike some of my compatriots who remembered everything, felt nothing, and talked to the operating crew (or thought they did) through the entire procedure.

Back in Miami, confronted with piled-up junk mail and enough shop-by-mail catalogues to stock an Antarctic expedition, I took a couple of days to orient myself to the changed geography. Then, no more stalling. I called Cy. I admit Anne joined in persuading me. She was ready for the curative procedures to get underway. With my concentration on my own insides, I was slowly beginning to realize the concern, and the preoccupation, of my family with my condition.

In his office, the day before I went to the hospital, Cy installed a catheter, a tube of slick plastic material, through my penis and into my bladder to drain the urine I had been storing as though it were something valuable. Actually, the amount had increased while I'd been up in the hills. I'd never had a catheter stuck in me before, especially in that particular organ. It was inconvenient, with its plastic bag hanging down to catch the drainage. It was awkward but not painful. It went in slick and easy. Obviously, the urethra, not to mention the penis itself, is a rather flexible tube.

The catheter has a little balloon on the end that fits into the bladder above the bladder neck and the sphincter there. The balloon is inflated with fluid so it remains in place like a little ball suspended above a socket, which is the bladder opening. The tip of the catheter extends out beyond the end of the balloon and the bladder drains through that extending tip. The balloon can't fit too tightly or it might damage the sphincter. The inflation of the balloon is adjusted so it stays where it is supposed to.

Came the morning. Events moved more swiftly. Off I went to Mt. Sinai hospital toting my overnight bag. Tests began speedily. Events moved more swiftly. I was not the first patient to be tested in this large hospital. They tested urine, blood coagulation rate,[2] chest xrays, everything they could think of. Nurse Helen Paulson, a large, handsome woman who could have been a Marine sergeant major, took charge of me. I wasn't intimidated but I had no intention of crossing her, either. Indeed, I couldn't think of anything to do but what she said to do. She was considerate and sympathetic but she was also boss.[3]

My wife Anne decided I required company or supervision or my hand held, or all three, so they moved a cot into my room and she became a participant. It was a good idea and her presence kept me from mulling about things to come.

A smiling young man entered the room. "Time for your shave," he said cheerily. "I don't need a shave," I said, "Thanks, anyway." "The doctor says you do," he replied, and proceeded to shave me from the upper thighs to the belly button and everything in between. I am a hairy person. Hairless, I was uncomfortably conscious that my various parts—thighs, intimate equipment—rubbed together when I moved, deprived of the cushioning effect of hair. I stuck to myself. I felt more naked than I felt simply with no clothes on. Being shaved is not all that uncomfortable, it's just a condition you are constantly aware of, and until the hair grows back several weeks later it reminds you that your anatomy has been tampered with.

In the late afternoon, after I had ingested about all the daytime TV even a hospital patient should have to take, the anesthesiologist and my "own" doctors came by. They looked at the chart, looked at me, said the equivalent of "hi, there!" and were gone. Well, the anesthesiologist did ask whether I was allergic to anything and if I knew any reason I should not have a local, spinal anesthetic. I didn't. I told him I didn't want to be knocked out completely and he said, "Oh, we'll just give you something to relax you before the spinal."

Did he ever! At 5:30 the next morning, they gave me a bourbon-shot sized drink of something plus one shot with a needle. I don't remember the spinal, the trip to the OR, the operation, or even that overworked hospital TV shot of ceiling panels and fluorescent light fixtures flashing past as I rode the trolley each way.

*   *   *

The TURP, Just What Does He Do in There?

With so many of us enduring the TURP procedure, I wanted to know precisely what the surgeon did inside the prostate itself. The following taped conversation, edited to eliminate duplication, gives a detailed review of my operation. More background and some of the detailed medical information is reported in part 2, chapter 25.

ME: *They gave me something to knock me out and it did. OK. Now I am lying on this table with my feet in stirrups, like I was going to have a baby. How many people were in the room?*

NASH: There's an anesthesiologist, also an anesthesiology fellow or resident; there's a nurse, she's the circulator. The surgery is a one-man job. I don't need another person to scrub or anything. The nurse is putting up bags of glycine, and changing the irrigation fluids. You are hooked up to IV (intravenous) fluids, irrigating fluid, and antibiotics. You might have another line into a vein, usually one. If you are a sickly patient you might have a central venous line and/or an arterial line. The irrigating fluid is for distension of the bladder and the operating area so I can see in there.

ME: *And how is all that fluid going in?*

NASH: The IV fluids go through the tubing from the hanging bags into a vein. The working elements are encased in a sheath, a rigid pipe that goes into the penis, and can go as far as the bladder. The sheath contains a resectoscope—that's the fiber optic light and lens that lets me see into there—and I have a little cutting tool. The tube with the irrigating fluid hooks up to a spigot at the end of the sheath, so the fluid flows through the sheath. The sheath is about the diameter of my finger. There is a wire at the end of the cutting tool that is attached to a spring-like mechanism that advances it and springs it back. An electrical current goes through the wire and cuts away pieces of tissue and cauterizes [*burns the place where a cut has been made, in order to cause the blood to clot (coagulate), to stop bleeding*].

ME: *And there's another loop that cauterizes?*

NASH: The same loop; there's only one loop. I have foot pedals. One pedal

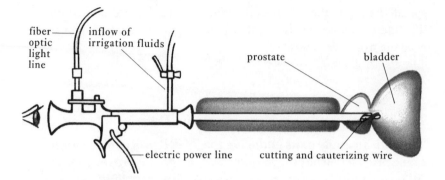

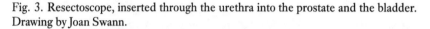

Fig. 3. Resectoscope, inserted through the urethra into the prostate and the bladder. Drawing by Joan Swann.

is for cutting and one is for coagulation and I can blend the two. I can have pure cutting, pure coagulation, or a blend, whereby I can cut and coagulate.

ME: *The cauterizing wire, does that mean there's a lot of blood?*

NASH: Some people bleed more than others. It also depends on how deep you are. The deeper you go into the prostate the more veins and arteries are cut. Anatomically, certain areas of the prostate have more blood vessels than others. There're certain areas where if you go beyond the capsule, you're into fat, the blood vessels retract and there could be more bleeding. You have to use a glycine irrigating solution in there that doesn't disperse the electric current. If you use saline (salt solution) you cannot cut. Glycine is a non-electrolytic solution, a mixture of sugars. With glycine you get no current dispersal.

ME: *Are there any risks using glycine?*

NASH: Even with the right solution, if you operate too long and too many vessels are open and the patient's absorbing all this fluid, he could become hyponatremic [*blood sodium too diluted*]. The systolic blood pressure goes up, the diastolic goes down, the pulse rate goes down, the patient starts to get agitated and then, if it progresses, he could get convulsions and die on the table. So the anesthesiologist has to check the pulse rate and the blood pressure and if there's any change that indicates fluid is being absorbed at too fast a rate, you've got to stop the operation and treat the patient. The post-op treatment would be fluid restrictions, diuretics by IV, and small volumes of "hypertonic saline," a 3 percent salt and water solution.

Now, a beginner may tackle too big a prostate and get a lot of bleeding, so the surgeon's experience about possible complications is important . . . with experience you can tell what's happening. Also the surgeon picks and chooses how big a prostate he can do safely. Some people can do a big gland safely: the manual dexterity required comes back to experience and training. Some try with too big a gland when they should have done a cut, an open subtotal prostatectomy [*an open incision into the prostate*].

ME: *How do you see with all this going on even with the fluids in the prostate and the bladder?*

NASH: We empty the fluid out occasionally. I'm in there and working. If the patient has a big bladder capacity it will hold the fluid and I keep on working. If he has a small bladder capacity, it'll only hold so much. How do I know when I have to empty the bladder? I know because all of a sudden it gets hazy in there. That means it's time for me to stand up and let all the fluid out with the blood and the tissue . . . let it out and start again.

ME: *You remove all the instruments then?*

NASH: No. I just take out the resectoscope, leave the sheath in. I take out the working elements and the fluid comes out through the sheath.

ME: *With all this going on in there how do you get out a piece of uncontaminated tissue for analysis?*

NASH: You mean for the pathologist? It comes out through the sheath with the fluid. It is not contaminated. I have a pan that the fluid flows through, the tissue remains. If the tissue is too big for the sheath, I use the loop and cut it into smaller pieces. That's the whole idea of the loop, that every piece I remove will come out through the sheath. At the end of the procedure, I scoop up all the tissue in the pan with a spoon, put it in a bottle of formaldehyde and send it to pathology.

ME: *OK. So now you are through with the operation.*

NASH: OK. Now I've cut out all the tissue that I'm supposed to; the patient hasn't required any blood; we give him antibiotics while we're working because there could be infection into the blood stream, so the patient is usually covered with antibiotics at the beginning and during the operation.

ME: *How long does the surgery take?*

NASH: I'm not including putting the patient under anesthesia and taking a look around. First you look into the bladder before you do the TURP. You cystoscope [*visually examine the bladder and urethra with the resectoscope*] to make sure there are no tumors or stones. Then you do your work. Depending on how much tissue you take out and how fast the

resection [*the actual cutting*] goes, it could be anywhere from thirty
minutes to an hour and a half. If it goes longer than that, you should
have done open surgery, unless the patient is too sick for that.

ME: *So this is a real operation, not like pulling a tooth?*

NASH: It's an operation with lots of possible complications and it can be
very dangerous in the hands of people who don't have good experience. Or it could be very simple. If the patient is medically stable and if
everything else is in order and goes fine, it's a piece of cake.

ME: *What do you do when you finish up?*

NASH: When we're all through, we've finished operating, we have to look in
and make sure all the prostate pieces are out. If there is a piece left
behind, that piece will block the catheter, or it can. We've got to make
sure that every little piece is out of the bladder and out of the prostatic
urethra. So we irrigate it using a couple of special instruments, and
make sure every piece is out. And then we look in again and when we
have to go back we cauterize all the bleeders because in removing all
these pieces with these instruments, we can set off bleeding again.

We cauterize or coagulate the bleeding points we can see just before we take the instruments out. And if it takes another ten minutes to
stop the bleeding we do it. As long as it takes. Then we take the instruments out and we put a catheter in, usually a large catheter, a three-
way catheter, a three-way Foley [*named for the person who developed the
catheter*]. Three ways, that is three tubes. One tube is to inflate the balloon that holds the catheter in place, the second tube is to get the fluid
out as you make urine, and the third is for a smaller inflow tube because we'll be irrigating the bladder continuously postoperatively. We
put a certain amount of fluid in to blow up the balloon [*to "anchor" the
catheter*] so that when we pull the balloon against the mouth of the
bladder we can stop any slight bleeding there that may continue after
the operation. And we've got to have enough fluid in that balloon. If
the balloon goes to the wrong place, if it pulls into the prostatic fossa [*a
sort of scooped-out place*] where we excavated tissue from the prostate
and if the balloon is pressing on the external sphincter, the patient can
be temporarily or permanently incontinent. So it's very important, that
the balloon, if it's a big resection, has a lot of water in it. If there is any
question about whether it pulls into the wrong place you just take it out
and put another one in. Very critical.

ME: *What do you do to prevent post-op incontinence?*

NASH: First, during the operation you avoid cauterizing or resecting too
near the external sphincter. Then, some people are incontinent after
the operation because the balloon pressed on the sphincter, inadver-

tently. There may not have been enough fluid in the balloon or the nurse or somebody pulled it too hard. So we usually then leave the patient on this traction with the balloon up against the mouth of the bladder, not in the prostate fossa but still in the bladder. That will keep the prostate cavity separate from the bladder cavity, so that any bleeding from the excavated cavity of the prostate will come out around the catheter.

The balloon is resting above where the internal sphincter was. That's gone, we remove that in the operation. So the only sphincter left is the external sphincter. So, therefore, beforehand a person had two sphincters, now after prostate surgery, he only has one, and the surgeon must protect that external sphincter.

ME: *OK, you're all through and the patient's sent to the recovery room.*

NASH: Right, and he's on traction overnight. Not everybody puts patients on traction, but I do it routinely. If there's not too much bleeding, we put them on little traction, a lot of bleeding a little heavier traction. The catheter with the balloon is strapped to the patient's leg, and the leg is tied down with the catheter emptying into a bag. So he's on traction till the next morning.

ME: *You call that traction.*

NASH: Right.

ME: *I thought traction was some guy with a broken leg. ["Traction" made me visualize legs in casts, suspended from pulleys over the bed, the slapstick view of an accident victim.]*

NASH: Put your penis on traction?

ME: *With a big weight on it.*

NASH: Right. Well, the next morning I call up and ask the nurse, "How's he doing?" and she says, "Well, everything looks good. There's not much bleeding." I say "Well, take him off the traction." So even before I get there, the nurse has him off the traction.

ME: *The catheter's still in but the pressure's off.*

NASH: The pressure's off. Then when I come in, if the patient has bladder spasms, the bladder doesn't like the catheter or the balloon, then where I had 60 or 70 cc in the balloon, I may drop it down to 20 or 10. And that plus a Benadryl shot will take care of a lot of the spasms. Then when the bleeding stops, when there's a day without bleeding, on the third or fourth day, whatever, then we take the catheter out.

ME: *Then after the TURP you have to wait at least seven or eight weeks if you're going to have any further surgery, any further action like radiation?*

NASH: Yes. We want the tissue to be healing along and want urination urgency and the infection and everything to be under control, because if there is infection or if you have urgency and frequency, it is going to be aggravated by the radiation, so we want a calm situation.

* * *

After the TURP

I returned to consciousness, no anesthetic hangover but groggy, in an intensive care postoperative recovery room. "Intensive care" is an oxymoron. I was monitored intensively by a machine and a few people who may have cared did drop by briefly. I discovered I was quite uncomfortable on a mattress far softer than my mattress at home or the one in my pre-operation hospital room. It was so soft it resisted any turning movement and I had to lift myself awkwardly to shift positions. Hospital attendants refused to concede the mattress was softer than any other. They probably figured I was still living, which was their primary concern, and that I'd be moved to a regular room the following day and, for one day, they had more to do than test every spare mattress in the place.

I had an ache in my testicles as though I were sixteen again and had been necking in a compact car for a couple of hours. It turned out I had *epididymitis*, an infection of the epididymides, small glands alongside the testes. This would take several weeks and heavy antibiotics to clear up. The lesson is, don't just lie there and hurt. Ask your doctor what's going on.

Lucky me! Epididymitis is a rare development in this era of antibiotics, Cy tells me. "We used to do vasectomies prior to TURPs. That kept infection from traveling to the epididymides. That's no longer usually done."

I dropped off to sleep about 8:40 p.m. but was awakened every two hours or so for temperature taking, blood pressure tests, and checks on an IV tube through which I was being administered antibiotics. Another suspended plastic bag fed a flushing fluid that flowed through the catheter into my bladder. There was a lot of action in the corridors and a jolly convention of nurses just outside my door though I couldn't quite hear what they were talking about. I had some shots to ease a nagging ache in my back, though this was the only postoperative pain I experienced. I still had a catheter, a new one, of course, and was on traction.

Also, I had a roommate, a gentleman who told me he had been a New York cabbie for thirty years. He fit the profile: friendly, loquacious, curious. Sometime during the night, my cabbie roommate suffered an attack of something that later turned out to be gas. He was in awful pain, screaming that he was dying. This caught the attention of the night crew who removed him, leaving me wondering what in the world happened to the poor devil.

He returned in the morning apparently all right. After my breakfast of cold eggs and some kind of wheat glue, the doctors showed up to marvel at my progress, evidenced by the fact that there was very little blood in my urine and I had almost no pain. Some minor pain can be expected, as well as possible bladder spasms and a strong desire to void. The balloon holding the catheter in place is inflated to 50, 60, or 70 cc, and is held in tension against the mouth of the bladder; when this "traction" is released, pain and spasms, if any, decrease. Your doctor may have to remove fluid and deflate the balloon to a smaller volume to stop spasms. My pain lasted a short time—a few hours—and I had no spasms, though I kept waiting for some to see what they were like.

I didn't remember in my entire life having any one evince so much interest in my excretory functions. I discovered I had lost any reluctance to discuss same and even went so far as to push information about my processes on doctors and nurses alike that certainly they could have gone without professionally. I felt like a two-year-old showing mommy what I had "made." I didn't know what was significant and what wasn't, however, and didn't want them to miss anything. They did seem interested. They cautioned me not to strain when performing my toilet chores.

We started changing rooms about 9:30 in the morning, and by 2:30 p.m. I was ensconced on the top floor with a brilliant view across central Miami Beach. I stood for about twenty minutes, had a minor discharge of blood into my bag, and through the afternoon received several floral offerings but no chocolate candy. A fellow in the hospital deserves at least a little chocolate since he is forbidden anything else not good for him. I suspected immediately that my wife and the medics had plotted to intercept any chocolate that may have been intended for me, and I planned to bribe some attendant to get me some from the hospital store, but I never found one subject to being suborned into chocolate smuggling. Besides, I realized I had no money with me. Advice: always tuck away a few bucks into a hidden compartment in your hospital overnight bag.

The recuperating patient takes special pleasure in small gains, remembering that much of the basic cancer that started all this rigmarole is still there multiplying its abnormal cells in its possibly fatal mission. My big gain was two days later: the catheter came out. To my enormous relief I could now move around without carrying my little plastic bag. I went to the bathroom like a real person.

Family physician Jim Furlong came around to check me out, commented that it was unusually early for catheter removal, looked at my chart and further commented, "You aren't very interesting."

Cy Nash, in and out in his quick way, cautioned me to watch for blood in the urine, to expect possible flashes of fever up to 103 degrees (they never happened) and some sweats as my body reacted to an invasion of infection following removal of the catheter.[4]

Except for the epididymitis, none of this happened. I remained on antibiotics. I felt fine, even took a walk down the hospital corridor and an elderly lady, seeing me pass, belligerently asked me what I was doing in her apartment. I told her it was a mistake, sorry. I even mooned Alton Road from my balcony, but not on purpose. The culprit was my ill-fitting hospital gown.

The next day, the third after the TURP, Cy gave me the first of two monthly shots of Lupron, the agonist that blocks testicular production of testosterone that fuels prostate cancer. Since I would wait at least two months before starting radiation treatments, so the TURP wounds could heal, he wanted to halt the cancer in its tracks. This is called "partial androgen ablation."

The Lupron, despite possibly causing an initial flare of a week or so in the cancer's activity when it is first injected, blocks the pituitary's signals to the testicles, stopping testosterone production and usually checking growth of the cancer cells. It is the hormonal equivalent of castration. To check a Lupron flare in the cancer, it may be necessary to administer an antiandrogen such as flutamide (trade name Eulexin) before a dose of Lupron. The flutamide blocks cancer cells from utilizing testosterone from the adrenal gland and other sources that increase their output when testicular androgen is shut down. As Lupron wears off in twenty-eight to thirty-three days, my radiation treatments were planned to start about thirty-five days after the second shot. Radiation is thought to be more effective when the cancer cells' activity is not suppressed. I felt some hot flashes a few times, nothing pronounced, and except for a certain bitchiness recognized no other effects from the Lupron. The shot is in the buttocks.

The worst pain is the cost, $492 a shot, of which if you are eligible Medicare pays 100 percent. I had a passing thought that it is somewhat outrageous that Medicare assigns a fee limiting what doctors should receive while pharmaceutical manufacturers charge what they please and get it. There's an alternate drug, called Zoladex, about $100 a dose less expensive, that is equally as effective as Lupron.[5]

If complete androgen ablation is a person's principal and protracted treatment, he will have either an orchiectomy, which means surgical removal of the testicles, or he will be on Lupron or Zoladex the rest of his life, plus, probably, a drug like flutamide. Meanwhile, I stayed on antibiotics, now Vibramycin, and two days later, a five-day total stay, departed Mt. Sinai and went home.

Cy advised me to wear a jock strap, even while sleeping, to ease the weight of my aching balls, slowly improving with the medicine. The infection finally eased some thirty days after the TURP, about par for this problem. Jim Furlong said it was all right to play golf. Cy Nash said I could putt. Of course, someone had to quip that the operation must have been wonderful because I never could putt before it.

As I began to circulate in the city once again, I met more and more men who had been through the same drill. There is little distinction in bearing this disease; it is too common. As I progressed, I had no residual pain. I had some constipation from the Vibramycin antibiotic, but that cleared up when I stopped taking the stuff and my bowels soon became as normal as they ever were. Follow-up visits with Urologist Nash continued. He advised against excessive physical exertion but I did play a few rounds of golf, as badly as ever. I continued to write my column for *South Florida* magazine and for the newspaper in Gainesville, Georgia, activities good for my morale. I continued to read and study about prostate cancer, slowly learning to translate medical books and articles into more familiar language. I said to Anne one evening, "You know, this is kind of scary. I just read this really technical article and I think I understand it."

Now Nash and Leonard Toonkel, M.D., chief oncological radiologist at Mt. Sinai, began preparing me for the linear accelerator.

Within two weeks of my TURP I returned to an almost normal schedule of urination, getting up only once during the night and producing a strong stream, as though I were twenty again. I was sleeping four hours at a stretch, a luxury. I felt as though a couple of dozen years had fallen off my system. The urethra relining becomes the lining of whatever cavity remains in the prostate after the TURP, but I felt nothing different as that process progressed.

In general, I felt considerably better than I did before the TURP, and people said I looked better, quite an achievement for medical science in my case.

Patient Meets the Ray Gun
Will I Glow in the Dark?

**. . . longterm survival after irradiation diminishes
systematically with more advanced disease, but it does not fall
to zero even in the most advanced stage.**
MALCOLM A. BAGSHAW, M.D., and colleagues

BY "NOT FALLING TO ZERO" Dr. Bagshaw means not all irradiated patients
with seriously advanced disease will succumb to prostate cancer. It will
work sometimes even on the worst cases. Men with localized cancers
(stages A and B) score survival times equal or almost equal to nonafflicted
men of their age group in the general population.

Radiation comes in two main categories: "external beam," meaning
xrays fired from a linear accelerator or other source outside the body, and
brachytherapy or "implants." The next chapter deals with implanted radioactive "seeds." Because your physician will want you to participate in
your treatment decision, you should be aware how each of these procedures, and surgical therapies, also, works. The upsides and downsides of
each are expanded upon in the "treatment choice" chapters later on.

Radiation technology is improving with better CT scanning and "lo-
calization" techniques. Newer methods of boosting effectiveness without
stretching safe limits of dosages are expected to increase external beam
(XRT) benefits. But even with capsule-contained tumors—A's and B's—
the possibility of recurrence of the cancer after radiation is high enough to
warrant serious consideration of surgical removal of the prostate, if you are
otherwise qualified.

Also, because of danger of injury to the rectum and the bladder from
XRT, the LINAC's (LINear ACcelerator—of xrays) maximum dosages of
7,000 rads probably can't be taken any higher than they are now.

My own experience was with the accelerator so, naturally, let's examine that method first.

Here was my prescription for radiation by the linear accelerator at Mt.

Sinai Medical Center, as ordered by Dr. Leonard Toonkel, head of radio-therapy:

4500 v Gy in 25 fx to prostate & lower pelvic nodes
+2380 c Gy in 13 fx coned down to prostate only, 4 field box technique on high energy linear accelerator

This meant twenty-five days of zaps over a fairly wide area, hip bone to hip bone, at a certain level of strength, which I later learned was about the usual; followed by 13 days of zaps focusing (coned down) to the prostate area only. These were about the routine dosage and pattern for a patient with my assorted xray, CT scan and other readings, and cancer stage. It is a substantial amount of radiation and if my tumors should recur, external beam radiation will not be used a second time to the same area because of fear of damage to healthy tissues. A few years ago, when irradiated seeds (brachytherapy) made a major advance in technique and technology, re-searchers hoped they would be effective agents for use in cases where initial treatment with external beam radiation had not been successful. Unfortunately, subsequent studies have demonstrated that seeds are not effective as a salvage procedure after external beam failure.

Frank Lake, M.D., oncological radiologist at Northeast Georgia Re-gional Medical Center in Gainesville, who became my advisor when I was away from Miami and Dr. Toonkel, tutored me patiently: a given organ can take only a certain amount of radiation and it "always remembers." The lungs, prostate, rectum, bladder, each has a tolerance level and can take only so much. Once an area has had, say, 6,500 to 7,000 rads of xray energy any more at any time risks complications. Radiation in some other region of the body would be permitted and there are some exceptions to all these statements.

Nothing in medicine is 100 percent. Yet, in this age of the bomb every grammar school child knows that radiation overdoses are dangerous.

Dr. Toonkel's prescription followed a couple of hours devoted to "lo-calization." This is the process of aiming the rays from the linear accelera-tor for maximum effectiveness for each individual patient. It requires a CT scan of the pelvic area and some additional xrays. Technicians went through this drill briskly. They marked spots on the right and left side of my frontal pelvic area with dots of indelible ink. There still wasn't much hair there after my pre-TURP shave two months previously. They drew indelible ink cross marks where my thighs join my trunk and cautioned me not to wash them off. Of course, they did wash almost off, but in the course of daily treatments were redrawn.

The information obtained during localization resulted in computa-tions by the doctors and a physicist who derived the prescription. They also designed a "block," a chunk of alloy weighing four or five pounds shaped to shield specific areas of my body from the accelerated rays. Every patient has a somewhat different block.

The radiologist draws a diagram for the block. His intention is to make sure that treatment hits where it is needed and that other areas are shielded from radiation. Calculations by a physicist and technologists help fix the precise shape of the block. Mine was a lopsided cube about six inches on each side with some curvature on each surface. This block is attached to a clear plastic base about an inch thick and a foot square. The block mechanism fits over the "lens" of the LINAC machine to provide for the patient's personalized pattern of intense xray exposure.[1]

What was a couple of hours for me involved considerably more preparation time by physicians, technologists, and physicists. This is Ph.D.-level work. Dr. Carlos Perez at Washington University, after a series of anatomical studies, developed methods of identifying the location of the prostate gland and seminal vesicles. With information from the CT scan, using as general benchmarks such reference points as the bony structure, hip bones, and the hip joint, where the large bone of the thigh (the femur) goes into the pelvis, a treatment-planning computer program simulates the radiation pattern with the CT's film. The extent of the seminal vesicles is also determined and this suggests the vertical reach of future radiation. With the fluoroscope, using a contrast medium in the bladder, the front and rear extent of the subject area is defined. In modeling the treatment, the computer actually places the radiation beam on the CT image. The dosage may be calculated. Much of this planning follows fairly standardized procedures, but these techniques allow individual planning for the differences from one patient to another. The eventual zaps from the LINAC will be set to allow some treatment adjacent to the target area in order to hit stray cancer cells, if any.

Later, when I went into the room containing the machine I saw several blocks lying in a corner on the floor awaiting their customers. OK, I thought, no reason to keep them sterile; they don't touch anyone and the rays they pass should kill any infectious organism smaller than a palmetto bug.

All this background planning and manufacturing may help explain why radiation treatments run about $130 a day, for about one full minute of exposure per day. Depending on its size and strength, the linear accelerator itself costs from $600,000 to as much as $1,200,000.

By this time, in the early part of the fourth month of my confrontation with prostate cancer, my prior and ordinary interest in the science and technology of medicine expanded congruent with my vital personal pursuit of survival. Yet I went through the technical details with a sense almost of detachment. I knew vaguely what the technicians were doing, but I couldn't affect the routine one way or the other. I did all I knew to do, which was to submit passively as the dispassionate object of their ministrations, which they carried out with close attention and some dispatch.

My localization complete, I collected my special parking pass for a space near the door of the radiology department, was instructed by one of Toonkel's colleagues to eat what I pleased but avoid too much roughage and not to swim. "Chlorine in the water may irritate your skin because it may become sensitive to the radiation," he said. I forgot to ask about swimming in the ocean, but in twenty-four years in Miami I haven't been to the beach a single time. Most Floridians don't swim in the ocean: that's for snowbirds (tourists and winter residents). The Floridians snorkel or scuba dive off the reefs or in the Keys. I went home with my marks, to my pamphlets on prostate cancer and my borrowed urology journals, plus some new material from the National Cancer Institute to await my role as a target in the medical Stars Wars script. (For details and background on the technology, see part 2, chapter 28.)

Meanwhile, I delved deeper into what I might expect in the way of a "cure," and pondered the possible effects of the rays on my body.

Now, candidates for definitive radiation as an initial treatment will have A1, A2, B, and C staged tumors, with careful evaluation of the C's for distant metastases. In the late 1980s, medical writers generally agreed with studies that showed that radiation and surgery were about equal in five-, ten-, and fifteen-year survival studies, with allowances for the greater selectivity involved in patients subjected to surgery. More recent presentations strongly support surgery for capsule-contained tumors, when it is feasible, as promising a higher percentage of disease-free follow-up and a lower incidence of recurrence of cancer as indicated by elevated PSA readings and biopsies.[2]

I noted in my homework that only 5 or 6 percent of irradiated patients suffer aftereffects necessitating hospital treatment, and that out of some 1,400 cases in one major study, only one died as a consequence of treatment. We seem to have about a 50–50 chance of preserving potency after radiation. Dr. Stephen N. Rous, author of *The Prostate Book*, uses 50 percent as a figure for permanent impotency, and Dr. Ruben F. Gittes, of the Scripps Clinic and Research Foundation, in a comprehensive review of prostate cancer, quotes Dr. Bagshaw's group's study of 532 patients which found that 86 percent retained potency after fifteen months and 50 percent remained potent after seven years.[3] The "ray gun" seems to involve nerve conductivity more than the blood vessels that engorge the corpora cavernosa (chambers on either side of the penis) and cause an erection. Even when some potency is retained, diminution can be expected over time.

Some other side effects of radiation, what the docs call "morbidity," are possible, principally irritations of the colon and other organs, cellular inflammations, and the like. About 10 percent of patients develop proctitis—bowel problems—of varying degrees and duration; there may be short-term fecal incontinence. Sometimes there may be some irritation of the small intestine, some burning when urinating, or mucus in the stool. Perhaps a given patient will find that one effect dominates or that there are no side effects at all. In severe instances, these problems could become chronic. In those patients who have had TURPs, some stricture of the urethra may occur. Not to give away the plot, but I had none and the rate of these problems is in the single digits percentage-wise.

I had a quick visit with Dr. Nash for a preradiation checkup. I still had a tad of epididymitis remaining but otherwise was OK and cleared to proceed.

Day One of the Zap Routine

I chose radiation over surgery for several reasons. One was, I didn't want to go through an operation because I dread being knocked unconscious and didn't want the long recovery experience. Another was that Cy Nash seemed to think radiation suited my needs and mindset, plus the suspicion that I might be a borderline C and could have some microscopic cancer cells outside the prostate. Another was that I live within a ten-minute drive of the hospital, an easy daily commute for the thirty-eight mornings I would have to trek back and forth through traffic. My usual golf course sits between the hospital and my home.

I arrived with my ink marks intact and was directed toward a waiting room with small changing booths attached. The hospital wants the patient in one of its gowns. They let me keep my shoes on but everything else had to come off. There is a certain leveling influence of the gown but although the waiting room contained about ten people in various stages of repair all of us watched some stupid morning show on the TV and did not talk to each other, even the ones who had been attending the place for several days, even weeks.

I was satisfied with the silence. I didn't want to talk about my cancer. The others may have had far worse disease than I. They weren't hostile; they were merely wrapped in their own thoughts plus those gowns that you know gap open shamelessly in the rear. I stuffed my street clothes in a flight bag and waited.

At exactly the appointed time, my name was called and I walked into a room with THE MACHINE.

The entry hall formed a zig-zag, almost a perfect Z, so no rays could escape it. Most of the machine's works are behind another wall. I saw them later, a huge block of boxes with wires, similar to the radar equipment room on a ship with several radars. What I saw in the large room was a sort of wheel vertical in the wall. Attached to its rim was a six-foot protuberance maybe a foot and half in diameter clad in cream-colored plastic. At the end of the projecting tube was the lens for the rays. My personal block was fitted over the lens. I knew because it had my name on it. The name on the machine itself was "Toshiba." They've caught up with me at last, I thought, one on one, *mano y mano*, but no kamikaze this time. The machine was certainly in no danger from me. I learned later that LINACs are also made by American firms.

The technicians in the room greeted me cordially, politely turned aside any attempt at conversation, especially my weak jokes about Japanese futuristic technology. "On the table, please," they said. I clambered onto a table that situated most of my posterior over a glass plate. Of course, the table was narrow and I had to lock my arms over my chest. They put pillows behind my head and maneuvered the lens of the LINAC into position, placing it about a foot from my body.

"Back in a minute," they said, and left the room. The controls they use are outside the Z corridor to protect the technicians from exposure. I waited. Shortly, I heard a loud hum as the machine warmed up and then emitted a more strident buzz for about fifteen seconds. The technicians returned and rotated the arm of the LINAC so the lens was completely under me, focused on my lower back. The technicians departed again; again the hum and the brief buzz. The procedure was repeated as they zapped me from each side, rotating the arm into the proper position. I guessed not more than a minute of zaps, in total.

"Is each exposure about fifteen seconds?" I asked. "We don't watch the time," they replied. "We set it for the dosage."

That was it. I felt nothing. No heat. No tickle. Nothing. I never throughout the thirty-eight days felt any sensation whatever from the LINAC.

My diary reports that on the fifth day there still was no specific reaction. By the fifteenth, I developed a marked bloated feeling and my waist went from its usual 38 to about a 42. None of my britches fit and I pushed my belt below my tummy like a country sheriff. I was warned of possible diarrhea but again I had none at this point. My principal problem was insomnia, especially after my 3 a.m. stumble to the bathroom. My trips increased in frequency as the treatments continued, just when I had been regaining some control following the TURP. Normal, they said. Improvement began when the treatments ended.

The hospital dietician dropped by at an appointed time, said she wanted me to avoid any weight loss (actually I gained about five pounds) and avoid any fibers in my diet if diarrhea showed up. That was it. I had a scheduled weekly interview with a doctor on the radiological oncology team. He asked me how I was and I said fine except for the bloating. He went "hmm."

By the twentieth day, I did develop a mild diarrhea and was given Lomotil, shortly thereafter changed to Immodium, a patent drug slightly less strong. I had some swelling of the testicles, slightly painful. This receded after rest. Dr. Nash advised me to wear a jock strap but placed no restrictions on exercise. Also weekly the radiologists xrayed me to check on the proper aiming of the LINAC. My brother invited me to go fishing in the Keys for a few days and the doctors approved a long weekend, no problem. (It was windy as hell and we caught zilch.)

By this time, I was feeling the mild fatigue that had been forecast and had gotten used to donning my gown, sitting in the waiting room with my dour fellow sufferers and reading in order to escape the banal stuff on morning television. Where do they find those weirdos they interview? New patients came and went. They all looked forlorn in those gowns. I shared the waiting room for several visits with a young woman who had a disfiguring tumor on her face near her nose. I could see that it was growing smaller day by day. I hope she's cured, now. A few men about my age were there. I didn't ask them and they didn't ask me if we were brothers of the prostate but there was nothing visibly wrong with them.

The treatment visits took about an hour a day portal to portal. The remainder of the time went as usual, unaffected by the radiation routine. My reading about prostate cancer increased and I noticed a sudden increase also in the attention television news, magazines, and newspapers paid to the subject. Prostate cancer was moving out of the shadows. About this time various prominent people revealed their prostate cancers to the public: Broadway producer Joe Papp and Time-Warner chief Steve Ross, whose cancers proved fatal, and U.S. Senator Bob Dole, among others.

I was pretty well locked into Miami during the January through March course of treatment, didn't fly the airplane and, of course, couldn't take off long enough to get up to the hills. Eventually, the final day of zaps arrived, everyone at the hospital bid me farewell and good luck, and Dr. Toonkel said he'd see me in about three weeks. That checkup proved satisfactory to him.

About three weeks later Dr. Nash took another PSA test which showed a reduction from my 14 ng/ml prior to radiation down to 2.3 ng/ml, an unusually rapid decline. The preradiation Lupron and my TURP may have contributed to that. Very encouraging.

Between the test and the result thereof I flew up to Georgia where my grandchildren were visiting the mountain house. They had taken the message of the test results and knew them before I did. I landed in Gainesville and drove up the sixteen miles to the house. Taped to the garage wall was a sign painted by a four-year-old and a seven-year-old, in various colors of marker crayon with letters of assorted sizes. It said, unevenly, "PSA 2.3." A nice greeting.

Within three or four weeks of the end of the radiation course my urination schedule returned to the same frequency as it had been before any of this began. I was getting up once a night some three or four hours after turning off my reading light and again in the early a.m., about awakening time, anyway.

The PSA Drops

Anne and I launched into a summer of flying, private and commercial, an Alaskan cruise, and the general indolence of a couple supposed to be retired from daily labors. It was enough. I was glad to return to the hills and work on this book. I had carried several items of urological lore on our trip and by this time had a fairly clear concept of what I wanted to write. (That's a laugh. I didn't know what I was getting myself into.)

Then, about five and a half months after the end of the radiation course I returned to Miami and a Nash check-up, including a PSA test. The test reported a new low level of 0.6 ng/ml.[4]

Just to counteract any false euphoria—to wax too cheerful is to challenge the gods—I reminded myself that after time the PSA can start back up again if the cancer recurs.[5] Perhaps this attitude was a hangover from newspaper work. News people never really learn to handle good news well.

It goes almost without saying that I wanted particularly to study reports on the survival rates of irradiated patients and what progressive PSA readings might mean. Indeed, I found survival time might be more related to one's Gleason score—longer life with scores of 6 or less—than PSA. We'll examine all this when we get into each of the treatment decisions, by cancer stage. Also some stats on this are in part 2.

For what it's worth, I suppose the main lessons I can pass along from my radiation treatment are that (1) you won't glow in the dark, and (2) cancer cures aside, the odds are good you'll feel no discomfort and no serious aftereffects.

They Can Plant "Seeds" in You

Laying Radioactivity Directly on the Tumor

**The notable lack of rectal complications, particularly in the
combined treatment group, attests to the accuracy and reliability
of permanent implantation by this method.**
DR. JOHN C. BLASKO, on closed transperineal radioactive implants

WHAT'S HAPPENING AS TECHNOLOGY and knowledge increase is that the
long-time treatment methods for contained prostate cancers (and for BPH,
as we have seen) are being challenged by rapidly developing optional
methods. Principal among these are radioactive implants, familiarly called
"seeds," and "prostate freezing," which we'll talk about in the next chapter.

Insertion of radioactive materials into the prostate, medically termed
brachytherapy, probably started about 1911 when a Dr. Pasteau inserted radium using a catheter through the urethra.[1]

Early trials using radium produced a high percentage of complications. But the development of new "interstitial implant therapy" techniques and improved radioactive materials stimulated new interest as well.
If the implanted radioactive seeds work well, they may avoid some of the
problems of recurrence marking external beam radiation (XRT). Also, because of danger of damage to the rectum and bladder from XRT, maximum beam dosages are at their upper limit. Adding implants can almost
double the radiation strength without the concurrent damage to nearby
healthy tissues.

Dr. Porter told a San Francisco conference that several thousand patients have been treated with implants. So a record is building to assess the
effectiveness of the procedure. Its advantages over XRT and surgery include reduced cost to the patients, a very short stay in the hospital, if any;
quick resumption of normal activities, including sex, in most treatments;
reduced radiation risk to medical personnel and reduced possibility of
damage to prostatic adjacent tissues and organs. Time and the accumulation of statistics will judge.

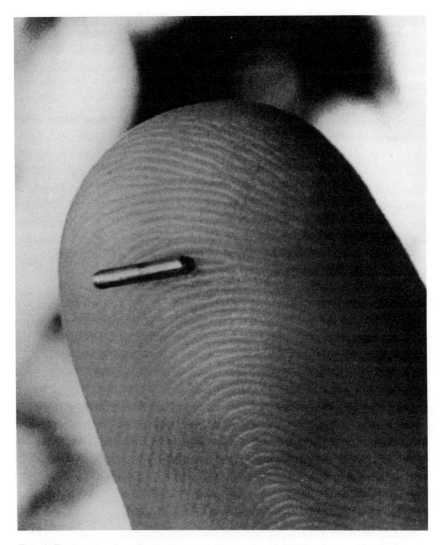

Fig. 4. Radioactive "seed" on a fingertip. Photo courtesy of Amersham Healthcare.

Techniques improving interstitial implants include the use of trans-rectal ultrasound in placing the seeds precisely, in a pattern designed to make sure all cancerous tissue is bombarded with radioactivity and finding and developing a variety of materials from which to make the seeds. In some instances, external beam treatment may be augmented by permanent seed implantation.

"Seeds" look like just that, seeds; like the seeds on rye bread, for example, or small grains of rice. With transrectal ultrasound guidance the seeds are put into place through needles inserted in the prostate. To be effective, they are set from 0.8 to 1 cm (0.32 to 0.4 inches) apart from each other in a three-dimensional grid. Since they don't shoot their radiation very far they do not endanger sensitive tissues elsewhere. Fifty to a hundred or more seeds might be inserted in the prostate, depending on the size of the prostate itself and the dose to be delivered.

At about $25 per seed for iodine-125, for example, this is not bargain basement treatment. Other elements cost more, palladium-103 about twice as much. Brachytherapy does cost considerably less than surgery or external beam radiation treatment, however. A smaller gland will require fewer seeds, but could require a higher strength dose per seed. Dosage is calculated to fit each patient. Seeds are prepared to the radiation strength the ordering physician designates by firms that form and irradiate the material. Seeds are inserted in the patient the day after they arrive from the "seed factory." The grid to help aim the needle through which the seeds are placed appears on the ultrasound screen.

The insertion access is perineal (between the scrotum and the anus). This approach seems to work better than the earlier used retropubic (from the front). That way involved open surgery, which caused its own complications and precise distribution of the seeds proved more difficult.

Seeds might be used as initial treatment, or in treatment of a recurring cancer. They might be used in conjunction with androgen blockade. They are frequently used in conjunction with external beam radiation when bulky tumors are involved, so the dosage at the tumor site can be stronger. Either open dissection of lymph nodes or a laparoscopic exam of the nodes may be necessary before seeding, to see if the cancer has spread.

Most implants being used now are permanent. The needle is withdrawn and the seeds remain. When their job is done, they stay in place. Some are temporary. These emit higher energies and higher dosages and usually employ an irridium isotope. They remain in place two or three days and are removed in a second procedure.

Drs. John Blasko, Peter D. Grimm, and Haakon Ragde of Seattle noted that advances in noninvasive imaging, radioisotope development, and computer-based dosimetry now allow far more accurate planning and execution of implants.[2] They use iodine-125 or palladium-103 either as a sole treatment or as a boost following 4,500 rad doses of external beam radiation for larger tumors. The isotope and the XRT dosage depend on the stage and grade of the offending tumor; usually Gleason scores of 2–6 received I-125 and those of 7 or higher Pd-103. Tumors staged as A, B0, and B1 are treated with implants alone and larger B2's with combined implants and XRT. With higher grade and stage lesions, especially if the PSA exceeds 20 ng/ml, lymph node examination may be required. They do not feel permanent implants should be used on C stage tumors and advise against using "seeds" on patients who have had a TURP, because of a higher incidence of incontinence.

Dr. Blasko and associates insert their implants on an outpatient basis under spinal anesthesia. Seeds are guided into predetermined positions with ultrasound. Some doctors use CT scanning and or fluoroscopy depending on their respective skills and preferences. All these methods are reported to work well.

Over six years, ending in 1991, Dr. Blasko and his co-authors reviewed results on several hundred patients. They scored a 93 percent rate of PSA return to normal levels (less than 4.0 ng/ml) and tallied clinical evidence of failure in 5 percent. The tests were too recent to attempt long-range survival statistics. Side and aftereffects were not excessive, but almost all the patients had irritation of their urinary system, urinary frequency, and some obstruction and urgency during the time the seeds emitted radioactivity (three to six months depending on which isotope was used).[3] Only one patient, who had had a TURP, suffered from long-term complications of the urethra and incontinence.

They reported a high degree of patient acceptance of the procedure and found the early, favorable PSA response encouraging. "In this era of cost containment, implant alone offers the potentially least morbid, fastest and least expensive method of treatment for early stage prostatic carcinoma," they said.

In a limited number of comparison studies, made of reports covering different time periods, implantation showed improved reduction of PSA counts over external beam therapy. In a comparison using a small study of surgical patients two years after treatment, implantation appeared almost equal in restraining PSA elevations.

Drs. Stanley Brosman, urologist, and Kenneth Tokita, radiologist, of St. John's Hospital and Health Center, Santa Monica, Calif., in correspondence with Dr. Nash, sent us a copy of their patients' information sheet, quite clear counsel for the man preparing for implants. They test for patient eligibility for the process to assure that the cancer is localized to the prostate and also schedule a pretreatment planning session at which they measure the prostate volume by ultrasound and design the grid indicating where seeds will be placed. A very large prostate might be rejected. If a large portion of the prostate is behind the pubic bone, implants may not be feasible. Sometimes the prostate can be shrunk with LHRH agonists, such as Lupron (see chapter on hormones), and in some patients the doctors elect to drill holes through the bone in order to place the needles. In some, angled needle placement is possible.

They want to know any medications the patient may be taking and they obtain the usual hospital pre-op tests, blood counts, an EKG, chest xray, and urinalysis.

They advise a light diet and order a laxative. An anesthesiologist talks with the patient. Usually, a spinal or an epidural anesthesia is administered. A catheter is inserted into the bladder. The patient is awake or dozing intermittently during the operation, they note. The implanting takes an hour and a half and afterward the patient goes to a recovery room. Two hours after the anesthesia wears off, he's ready to go home, clutching his antibiotic prescription and his recommendation that he take a stool softener. For a time, he is to avoid blood thinning drugs, such as aspirin or Persantine.

Depending on their type and strength, seeds go on working for an extended time, perhaps three to six months irradiating cancer and healthy cells alike as the patient goes about his business. The healthy cells can heal; the cancerous ones cannot, and slough off or are digested by the body. The recovery phase takes nearly a year, the doctors advise, which is why it takes so long to appraise the effectiveness of the treatment. They close their advisory with two comments of note: (1) the cost of the procedure is $10,000 to $12,000, including everything, and (2) sexual activity may be resumed within two to three weeks, or earlier.

Several days later Drs. Brosman and Tokita take xrays to check the dosage. In a 1991 report in *Urology*, they said their average number of seeds implanted per patient was 76.6, with 13 the low and 135 the high.[4] That's a lot of holes to punch in a man's crotch; no wonder it hurts for a week or so. But the discomfort is much shorter than that following surgery.

Consolidating several reports on implants, however, we found a minimum of consequential problems. The most common encountered by the Santa Monica team were bladder and urethral irritative symptoms in 90 percent, with 54 percent requiring medication for their problem. These symptoms abated within a month for most patients but some were troubled for four or five months. Of eighty patients in this study, five developed urinary retention and required catheterization for several days.

Other trials reported that there may be some swelling of the testicles for a short time and some urinary difficulties encountered. The chronic problems that appeared were with patients who had previous TURPs. Never say never in prostate cancer circumstances, but with TURP-treated patients, implants are approached with great caution, if at all.

The Brosman and Tokita patients experienced rapid decrease in prostate size and PSA levels. PSA's returned to normal or diminished more than 50 percent within six months among 97 percent of their patients.

In Miami, the Nash (urologist)–Toonkel (radiologist) team has strong hopes for seeds' efficacy. The pair has been building experience in the procedures. Dr. Nash measures the volume of the prostate, the radiological physicist determines the dosage (depending on the prostate volume) and the number of seeds to be used. In the urology operating room, Dr. Nash inserts the ultrasound probe and lines up the insertions on a grid. He inserts the needles and Dr. Toonkel loads the radioactive material—a team project.

The Miami team tried palladium seeds in treating recurrence of tumor after external beam radiation, as a salvage technique. The results looked good at first. Patient PSA's went down. But after eighteen months or so, some PSA's started to rise. At this point, the technique does not look promising for salvage therapy. Drs. Nash and Toonkel continue to use implants on selected patients but, as others, must wait for time to pass to gauge the long-term results.

Dr. Blasko and colleagues at the Northwest Tumor Institute reported on two treatment methods in response to our inquiry about their experiences. One group of patients was treated with iodine-125 or palladium-103, and another, with larger or more advanced lesions, was treated with external beam radiation followed by iodine-125 or palladium-103 implants. Complications were minimal, mostly from the insertion of the needles rather than from the radioactive material.

Dr. Blasko wrote, "Pain complaints have been surprisingly infrequent, with only ten per cent of the patients requiring any analgesic. Three patients (of 274) did experience significant perineal pain . . . following the implant which cleared up over several weeks without residual effects. Most patients resumed normal activities within 48 hours of the implant." The Blasko team studies have become the reference standard for this therapy.

In sum, for certain lesions, seeds seem to work better than external beam and, of course, they're quicker, since they take only one procedure. Seeds are also less expensive, although you don't want your treatment selected on a bargain basis.

Using seeds can save potency possibly 90 to 95 percent of the time. "If a patient wants to resume sex immediately, or if he wants to go fishing next week," Cy Nash said, "he might choose seeds over external beam therapy or even surgery. I had one fellow tell me, 'I want to keep living now. I don't want to worry about when I'm eighty. I'll take my chances on old age.' So treatment can also depend on where the patient's coming from."

In the relatively brief history of seeds' use in sufficient numbers to produce reasonable statistics on recurrence and survival in the several categories employed around the world, not enough time has elapsed for
comparisons with other therapies. Listening to the inner circle conferences of the urological world, you gather it thinks it isn't doing enough to
solve the mysteries of prostate cancer and to prolong the lives of its victims.
Interstitial implants, when the numbers are in, could relieve some of the
doubts about radiation versus the enigmatic cell.

13

Cryosurgery
Very Deep Freeze for the Cancerous Prostate

A MAJOR TECHNICAL ADVANCE in the early 1990s introduced a new procedure for treatment of prostate cancer—freezing that offending member into submission with subzero temperatures. If totally effective, the freezing and thawing process changes the original cell structure of the prostate to a bundle of inert fibers.

Very quickly, doctors added the method, called cryosurgery, to what they term their "armamentarium," meaning their inventory of "armaments" to fight the cancer. They had seen it used with success against other cancers.

The advance came with the development of instruments to circulate liquid nitrogen (LN_2) through five small tubes inserted like needles into the prostate through the patient's crotch generally with no necessity for a surgical cut. Technically, the procedure is termed "transperineal percutaneous cryoablation."

Reports so far struck me as extraordinarily upbeat for this usually skeptical group of medical specialists. Dozens have attended short training courses at Allegheny General Hospital in Pittsburgh, Pa., where Drs. Jeffrey Cohen and Ralph Miller, urologists, and Dr. Gary Onik, radiologist, began using transrectal ultrasound to "see" the freezing as it actually takes place, in "real time," as they call it. Emory University Medical School, in Atlanta, scheduled courses once a month in early 1994. Several other major centers added experience to the general knowledge and by early 1994 upwards of two thousand procedures had been performed in this country.

There are several reasons for urology's contained enthusiasm. For one thing, cryosurgery has been used for a quarter of a century in dermatology, gynecology, and other areas, and has proven effective in treating otherwise inoperable liver cancers, for example, among other malignancies. Conversion to liquid-carrying probes instead of nitrogen gas enabled delivery of lower temperatures and more precise and effective control, thus opening the way to treat tissues deep within the body. Earlier cryosurgical procedures used open perineal and abdominal surgical incisions to get to the prostate. This meant more surgery-related aftereffects in addition to those caused by inadequate freezing.

Other reasons for the optimism are that cryosurgery takes only one to two hours, causes no significant blood loss and fewer side effects than other treatments, means only two or three days in the hospital, and costs about half as much as radiation or surgical prostate removal. Two or three days after treatment the patient may return to normal physical activities. And for those of us initially treated by radiation it has the unique capacity in that "armamentarium" to perform as a second or salvage therapy if the cancer recurs.

The device is made by Cryomedical Sciences, Inc., of Rockville, Md. They label it the "CMS AccuProbe" system. The system circulates liquid nitrogen through the probes. Each probe is individually monitored through a control console and the whole process is constantly observed through rectal ultrasound imaging. The temperature cast by the probes is minus 180 degrees Centigrade, cold enough and equal to about 270 degrees below zero Fahrenheit. It's plenty cold, though the patient feels no chill: he is anesthetized.

Handling the probes and the accompanying rectal ultrasound probe with a new CMS machine at Mt. Sinai Hospital at Miami Beach, Dr. Nash reported that though the patient felt no chill, his hands and fingers did.

Five probes, each three millimeters in diameter, produce an overlapping pattern of "iceballs" of four centimeters diameter each (about 1.25 inches or approximately the diameter of an old silver dollar). The quick-chilled cells in the prostate are dehydrated and shrunk. Ice crushes the cellular tissue. At minus 40 degrees C (roughly 100 below zero F) the cells are destroyed. The thawing process leaves cells or cellular fragments in what amounts to pure water from the melting. The body's electrolytes mix with the water, and the changing concentrations of the electrolytes theoretically add to the destructive effects of the freezing.

Some surgeons will urge on you, in the twelve hours preceding the freezing—to clean out your urinary system—four liters (!) of weak solution containing bicarbonate of soda, potassium chloride, sodium sulfate, and something called polyethelene glycol 3350. It tastes like water; it's the volume of the stuff that's difficult. The brand name is "Colyte." The nurses call it "golytely" but it will make you go heavily.

The freezing-thawing deprives the cells of oxygen carried in small blood vessels, and the body's immune system takes over. The destroyed cells are gradually absorbed by the body, as white blood cells work over

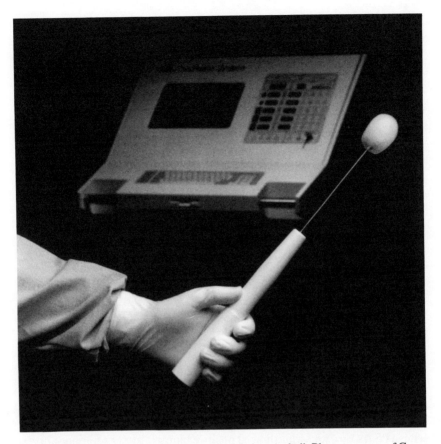

Fig. 5. Accuprobe console and Cryoprobe with 4 cm iceball. Photo courtesy of Cryo-medical Sciences, Inc.

many weeks, to leave behind merely fibrous tissue and no, or very little, tissue of the original gland.

The company received the patent for the AccuProbe device in 1991 when it solved problems associated with circulating the liquid nitrogen.

This is a fascinating method to me. One of my few early childhood memories is of a lecturer who came to an assembly of my grammar school when I was in the sixth grade. That was a very long time ago. He demonstrated liquid nitrogen by dunking a banana into a steaming container and then driving a nail into a block of wood with the frozen fruit. Boy, I thought, that's magic. Possibly still under the influence of a childhood impression, I found cryo-blasting to freeze somebody's internal organ selectively an em-inently reasonable tactic.

Since the frozen area can be finely controlled with ultrasound viewing and the probes, tissues outside the prostate, but close by, may be frozen or not as the operators desire. The probes can be inserted in the seminal vesi-cles. A urethral warmer is inserted through the penis and water from a heater is circulated at 37 degrees C (98.5F), or about normal body tem-perature. This protects the lining of the urethra and prevents freezing and damage to the inner lining of the voiding channel in the prostate. Minimal urinary incontinence has been reported so far. The probes are disposable after one use.

Cell structures vary as do sizes of prostates. In some men the prostate may be closer to neighboring organs than in others. It is possible for some cancer cells to elude the freezing probe. One of cryosurgery's advantages to the patient is that the treatment can be repeated without harm, a follow-up option not available with external beam radiation and, of course, not with surgery. Men treated with external beam have few options if the rays leave them, in a few years, with rising PSA's and possibly positive biopsies. Surgical salvage hasn't worked well. Radiation cannot be repeated. Only hormonal ablation with its unfortunate consequences and often limited period of effectiveness remains. And hormonal ablation doesn't cure; it merely holds cancerous progression at bay.

Cryosurgery may be the Lone Ranger riding to the rescue. At least two of the centers in their early use of the five-probe machine tried it on men whose PSA's rose and who showed positive biopsies after radiation. Short-run follow-ups (three to six months) revealed most PSA's down to the 0.3 ng/ml level. Positive biopsies placed the failure rate for the salvage process at 35 percent. Tests at other centers confirmed the greater difficulty of sal-vage cures following radiation. Later trials have produced better results. But if 65 percent of the men who fail radiation can be significantly im-proved, perhaps even cleared of cancer forever, the great scoreboard in the sky should light up and ring bells.

Dr. Timothy McHugh, St. Joseph Mercy Hospital, Ann Arbor, Mich., said in a communication to Dr. Nash that he uses Lupron for three months prior to cryosurgery to decrease the prostate size to 50 grams or less when necessary. He reported only 6 percent positive biopsy findings six months after primary treatment.

At the time of this writing, no long-term trials or comparative studies were available. Early judgments were made on the basis of rapid PSA de-clines and minimal aftereffects. After a year of following ninety-three patients, short run, Drs. Cohen and Miller reported 1 percent urge incontinence and 9 percent stress incontinence, considered probably controllable. A possible aftereffect could be bleeding, a 1 percent consequence in this report. Another possibility is numbness of the glans penis, the tip of the penis. The procedures found that 30 to 34 percent of those treated remained potent if they were potent prior to the treatment. Younger men retained potency more frequently than those over seventy. It is possible critical nerves may regenerate over time.

What are the other downsides? If the patient previously had radiation treatment the likelihood of incontinence increases, usually a temporary problem. Poorly differentiated tumors may not freeze as well as more differentiated ones. Failures, indicated by rising PSA's, might be caused by uneven freezing, or higher Gleason grade tumors might have more resistance, or perhaps there was tumor beyond the "freeze ball." Whatever. In the event of rising PSA's or positive biopsies they would wait six months and freeze again.

From the patient's point of view, the brief treatment time and lower cost make cryosurgery an attractive option. There is no pain during the procedure. Afterward the discomfort may exceed that of seed implantation because the holes punched in the crotch are larger; there may be some surgical cuts to insert the probes. These would be stitched closed.

An early report from three doctors at Allegheny General Hospital in Pittsburgh, Pa., working with Ph.D.'s from the University of California, Berkeley, Department of Mechanical Engineering, and from the manufacturer reported that of fifteen patients treated prior to 1 May 1992, fourteen (93.3 percent) showed no residual disease on short-term follow-ups. These figures reflected use of the five-probe system. Earlier trials with the previous two-probe system were not as successful. The doctors found total freezing wasn't taking place.[1]

This group reported a minimum of complications, some of which they blamed on inexperience with the procedure. None were serious. Of patients potent before the procedure, 35 percent were potent afterward. There may be some regeneration of frozen nerve tissue over time. One of their patients regained potency six months after his treatment.

In a previous report cited by the Allegheny group, the advantages of the process included the ability to treat patients with high stage disease, and with previous TURPs, the resulting minimal loss of blood, and a decrease in impotency compared with radical prostatectomies.

None of the Allegheny group patients suffered incontinence. One of their concerns was that freezing would extent to the rectum wall and cause *fistulas*, which are inadvertent connections between two or more functioning parts of the body, in this case causing urine leakage into the rectum.

They found they could add space between the prostate capsule and the rectum by raising the handle of the transrectal ultrasound probe, pushing the tip of the probe against the rear wall of the rectum, pulling it away from the prostate. So does science progress!

From mid-July 1992 to early October 1993, Dr. Andrew von Eschenbach and colleagues at M. D. Anderson Center, University of Texas, Houston, Tex., performed eighty-nine salvage cryoablations using the CMS AccuProbe. Dr. von Eschenbach, responding to a questionnaire from Cy Nash and me, said he considers the procedure an "excellent method of local tumor cell destruction" that may be "a suitable alternative to radical surgery or radiation for selected patients." However, through late 1993 the M. D. Anderson urologists were using it only as a salvage procedure for failed radiation patients and then only when they could confidently freeze all of the local tumor. They are following up with PSA tests monthly for six months, transrectal ultrasound at three and six months, and biopsies at six months.

Dr. von Eschenbach said that the procedure is generally well tolerated by patients, but for a subset of patients prolonged voiding problems may occur. He noted that the procedure requires exceptional skill at ultrasonography of the prostate.

He presented a paper to the 1994 annual meeting of the American Urological Association in San Francisco reporting on fifty-one patients with local tumor recurrence following radiation who received cryoablation at M. D. Anderson. Their average age was seventy, range sixty to seventy-eight. Biopsy confirmation of radiation failure showed a full range of tumor grades among the patients; twenty-two of them had Gleason grades of 8 or higher. Their recurrence occurred after a range of 10 months to 16.4 years. Forty-six had a PSA decline to less than 4.0 ng/ml after cryosurgery and in seventeen PSA became undetectable. Ten patients who had positive biopsies on follow-up (five of whom had only minimal disease) underwent a second cryoablation, but the results of those aren't in yet.

"Our data suggest this an ideal method of treatment for patients with local recurrence of tumor following radiation. . . . [It] has been well tolerated and over two-thirds have been initially rendered biopsy-negative in spite of the fact that their recurrent tumors were of advanced stage and grade," he reported.

If the procedure as an initial therapy generally produces a 93 percent success rate as it did for Drs. Onik, Cohen, Miller, and McHugh, it would be about the equivalent of surgery on a truly contained cancer and would compare more favorably with radiation with appreciably less risk of contrary aftereffects. "If that promise holds," Dr. Nash observes, "cryosurgery could replace the radical prostatectomy and external beam xrays in a substantial number of men." Such a result would change the world landscape of prostate cancer treatment.

But let us not get carried away. If two and five and ten years must pass in order to assess the permanency of an apparent cure, and another five to confirm a cure, cryosurgery remains in its statistical infancy. Nevertheless, at approximately $260,000 a unit, hospitals are buying AccuProbe systems as though they were "Quiet, Please" signs. As of September 1993 almost before the ink had dried on the patent, fifty hospitals had installed them, so there are now at least fifty-one because I know myself of one installed since then.

In the same issue of *Cancer* as the Allegheny team report, an editorial by Dr. Gerald W. Chodak of the University of Chicago said, in effect, cool it until we can see how this works over time.[2] Dr. Chodak probably would never stoop to such an obvious pun. What he really said was that more information is needed before the role of cryosurgery can be determined. "Another limitation is that no information is yet available on the failure rate or the short term and long term adverse effects over time. Also," he asks, "how will cryosurgery affect the efficacy and morbidity of subsequent radical prostatectomy or radiation therapy after cryosurgery if a complete response is not achieved. Longer follow up is needed."

Dr. Chodak, however, called it a potentially valuable therapy worthy of investigation. He noted the possibility of repeat procedures and the promise of delivering treatment outside the capsule and into the seminal vesicles where tumor frequently extends.

The Food and Drug Administration has cleared the AccuProbe for use in urology, oncology, general surgery, dermatology, proctology, and eye, ear, nose, and throat surgery. It is not a single-purpose device. But individual hospital leadership approval still is required for deep penetration use as in prostate cancer treatment.

By the time you read this, increasing applications of prostate cryosurgery may have altered the picture, but as I write, several major insurance carriers still regard the treatment as experimental and do not reimburse for percutaneous cryosurgical ablation so coverage and payments have been assigned on a case-by-case basis. The manufacturer says that more than thirty carriers, as of 1993, reimbursed for the procedure. It said a Medicare reimbursement code is in place for open transperineal and abdominal cryosurgical removal of the prostate. Since the percutaneous method is faster and cheaper, presumably the insurers are waiting only for more published professional confirmation of the procedure. This may have come to pass by the time you read this.

Several trials of cryosurgery on stage D cancers, when known meta-stases are present, are reported, seeking an immunological improvement, meaning they hope to weaken the tumor source and so diminish or prevent further spread. It has been applied to A2, all the B stages, and C stage patients. Since total removal of the prostate seems to have prolonged sur-vival in some patients who have stage D cancers with limited metastases, perhaps the iceballs can do the same. We'll have to wait to learn if it works for that, just as we will allow time to bring in more information on the gen-eral efficacy of turning our prostates into popsicles.

The Radical Prostatectomy
Get That Problem Out of There!

There is now strong evidence that radical prostatectomy is
superior to radiation in treating localized prostate cancer
. . . and increasing evidence that radiation therapy is not
nearly as effective as was previously believed.
CHARLES B. BRENDLER, M.D.

DR. BRENDLER'S ADVOCACY is well based. In your decision process, if you
are eligible for surgery, it must go on your scale. But read the radiologists,
too.

Brothers of the prostate seem willing to share their experiences. One I
talked to, a sixty-six-year-old Kansan, underwent what appears to be a
textbook case of a happy outcome, a strong affirmation of the benefit of
catching it early. On a routine physical, a DRE (digital rectal exam) yielded
no problems. This was later confirmed by a urologist. He also had a PSA
test. It showed a reading of 5.5, only a slight elevation. With a PSA of 4 to
10 there's a 20 to 30 percent chance cancer is present and DRE's can miss
them.

The urologist took six Biopty gun tissue samples, aimed by transrectal
ultrasound, and discovered tumor tissue of low grade in one of them. Although his doctors appeared to him reluctant to operate on a tumor as yet
so unthreatening (many would not be reluctant), my "brother" wanted it
out of there and did not want the consequences of radiation that had been
reported to him. (By today's medical consensus, he made the right choice
for his size tumor although some would "watch and wait.")

He underwent a three- to four-hour "nerve-sparing" radical prostatectomy (a technique developed to preserve potency) with a general anesthetic and was unconscious about eight hours. Lymph node sections
were biopsied after he was incised and showed no tumor invasion. He endured almost no pain and after he had used a patient-regulated pain killer
for one day, the IV analgesic drip tube he controlled was removed. His uri-

99

nary catheter was removed seventeen days after the operation, some four days under the average for such procedures. After that, he wore a diaper for about five days, switched to a smaller pad, and in about ten more days regained both confidence and urinary control. He exercised those muscles, he told me.

Two months after the operation he was working to return his golf game to its usual high-nineties level, walking a mile and a half on a treadmill at 3.8 mph, and even helping his son move to a new residence, lifting his end of a couch. He had not had a follow-up PSA when I spoke with him. His operational wound was still a little sensitive, but otherwise he felt OK and was looking forward to a future test of the "nerve-sparing" effort. That benefit would take some more time. This is an example of the best way this operation can go.

In a radical prostatectomy, the surgeon removes your prostate completely, and also the seminal vesicles that lie along the prostate. So, if your cancer has been staged accurately as totally capsule-confined and the surgeon knows what he's doing, there's a high chance the operation will rid you of the cancer for good. Your total medical expenses will range from about $15,000 to $20,000, depending on variations in hospital charges. This cost is in the neighborhood of total costs for external beam radiation, as well, perhaps a little less in some hospitals.

Most "radicals" are performed on localized cancers, that is, cancers judged to be confined to the prostate itself. These are specifically staged as A1, A2, B1, B2, and B3 tumors. In some of the surgical series reported, up to 60 percent of tumors staged as B2 could turn out at surgery, when the microscope can examine them later in the pathology lab, to be C and D1 tumors instead, meaning that some tumor had escaped the prostate capsule and some was found to an extent in the lymph nodes. Up to 20 percent of the clinical C's could prove at surgery to be downstaged to pathological B's.

As we've noted already, some surgeons are proceeding with the removal of the prostate even if they discover minimal invasion of the nodes and may follow up surgery with radiation treatments and/or orchiectomies or hormonal treatment, hoping to prevent recurrence. The chance for long-term disease-free survival isn't quite as good at these advanced stages as when the tumor is truly localized.

As recently as the early 1970s, radical prostatectomy was not undertaken enthusiastically by either patients or surgeons because it was technically difficult and carried a substantial risk of side effects, including serious blood loss and almost certain impotency, plus up to 10 percent postoperative urinary incontinence.

**Distribution of Treatment Methods by Clinical Stage of Disease
for Newly Diagnosed Prostate Cancer (Percentage)**

	Stage A		Stage B		Stage C		Stage D	
	1984	1990	1984	1990	1984	1990	1984	1990
Prostatectomy	6.5	10.1	14.7	27.5	4.1	10.4	.6	1.1
Radiation Therapy	16.3	16.5	40.0	40.6	38.5	36.1	7.8	5.8
Hormone Therapy	8.4	6.0	11.7	9.0	28.6	27.7	61.5	64.4
Combination	2.4	1.7	5.6	6.2	10.5	11.8	16.2	14.9
None	66.4	65.7	28.0	16.7	18.3	14.0	13.9	13.8
Total	100	100	100	100	100	100	100	100

This table shows the range of treatments for prostate cancer and which methods are most popular according to cancer stage. Note the increase in prostatectomies for stage C and earlier cancers as urologists became more convinced of the efficacy of surgery, while radiation usage remained fairly stable across all stages. Cryosurgery was not in general use in 1990. Source: 1984 and 1990 American College of Surgeons Commission on Cancer patient care evaluation studies. Reprinted from *Ca—A Cancer Journal for Clinicians*, March/April 1993 (used with permission).

Today it is a common treatment for early prostate cancer and is increasing in use because more and more men are being diagnosed earlier, thanks to the addition of transrectal ultrasound and the PSA test to the standard DRE. Thus more localized and operable prostate cancers are being discovered. Moreover, techniques have improved and knowledge of the anatomy of the prostate and its surrounding area has moved forward considerably.

Patrick C. Walsh, M.D., of the Johns Hopkins Medical Institutions in Baltimore, wrote in 1988 that "over the past 10 years, the morbidity [related ill effects] of the procedure has been reduced by lowered blood loss, improved operative exposure [with new procedures, surgeons can see their work better], reduced postoperative complications . . . and assured urinary control in virtually every patient and potency in most."[1]

Dr. Walsh, who is urologist-in-chief of the James Buchanan Brady Urological Institute at Johns Hopkins, reported in its prostate cancer *Update* newsletter an evaluation of six hundred men who underwent his "nerve-sparing" operation from one and a half to eight years previously.[2] The local recurrence rate at five years was 4 percent; distant metastases, 7 percent; and 3 percent died of the disease. Compared to other published records, Johns Hopkins's record is extremely good. Ten- and fifteen-year evaluations are planned when the years unfold.

Indeed, Dr. Walsh himself advanced the cause significantly in 1983

through detailed studies of the anatomy of the prostate and its environment and his part in the development of what is known as the "anatomical"
or "nerve-sparing" surgical method. His approach to surgery is retropubic, that is, through the patient's lower abdomen.

In this adaptation of former surgical techniques, he attempted to preserve either one or both of the bundles of nerves and blood vessels that lie
along either side of the prostate near the bottom of the prostate capsule. I
am deliberately courting some error here by avoiding the technical medical
terminology for this complex of vital services to that area of the body—and
to you. In any event, in the bundles are the nerve message paths and blood
vessels that energize and serve your erection. This operative technique
usually is reserved for younger patients (at least a ten-year life expectancy)
with less volume of tumor and in otherwise good health, and the "nerve
sparing" aspect always takes second priority to the removal of tumor itself.

The surgeons' primary objective is to get all the cancer out of there;
secondarily to preserve potency where practicable. Dr. Walsh's work established a sort of baseline for urology. Others' evaluations of surgical outcomes invariably include pre-Walsh and post-Walsh comparisons.

Dr. Stamey of Stanford and the Mayo Clinic group published various
modifications of the operation, as well, and Dr. David Paulson of Duke has
applied the nerve-sparing technique to perineal (incision through the
crotch) radical prostatectomies.

The nerve-sparing procedure also enables surgeons to operate in a
less bloody environment than previously by early ligation of the dorsal
vein complex (meaning tying off a group of veins early in the operation that
would otherwise release a lot of blood later as the operation progressed),
thus using less transfused blood (usually the patient's own, previously
taken and stored), to see better what they are doing, and to somewhat
shorten the time required.

In the 1991 report, Dr. Walsh categorized the postoperative sexual
function in 503 men who had the operation that preserved or excised the
neurovascular bundle(s) of their prostate:

> both nerves left intact: ages less than 50, 90 percent potent; 50–59,
> 82 percent; 60–69, 69 percent; and 70 or over, 22 percent;
> one nerve partially excised: less than 50, 100 percent; 50–59, 73 per-
> cent; 60–69, 50 percent; and 70 or over, 50 percent;
> one nerve widely excised: less than 50, 91 percent; 50–59, 58 per-
> cent; 60–69, 47 percent; 70 and over, no report.

Prospective surgical patients can be encouraged by this record,
though we must say that every surgeon may not have skills comparable to
Dr. Walsh's. He found the figures "exciting news" and looks forward to

techniques that might restore erectile function through nerve regeneration or possibly nerve grafts.

A Virginia friend, a professor at the University of Virginia (I suppose we are all of the age of prostate problems), underwent a radical prostatectomy by Dr. Walsh himself and, a year afterward, reported no postoperative troubles whatever. Dr. Walsh could save only one potency-controlling bundle. The patient's PSA fell to zero. The patient reported a slow return of potency and says he is "almost there, but not quite." He uses a vacuum device while waiting for time to return his prowess.

His prostate cancer saga began when a local urologist found nothing on a DRE about three years ago, then the following year felt a suspicious lump. A biopsy located a Gleason grade 7 prostate cancer. After his operation, the Virginian found a congenial club of brothers of the prostate in the hospital recovery area who enjoyed greeting each other, as they walked around with their drain bags attached, with such cheery salutations as, "Your urine looks very clear today."

Two Surgical Approaches

There are two approaches to a radical prostatectomy. One is "perineal," in which the operation is performed through an incision between the scrotum and the anus. This is somewhat faster and yields a faster recovery time but sometimes may require another procedure for lymph node analysis, usually performed before the prostatectomy and possibly by laparoscopy. Checking the lymph nodes is something you may find in the medical literature abbreviated to SPLND, or "staging pelvic lymph node dissection."

A three-person Duke University team of Drs. Harold Frazier II, David F. Paulson, and Judith E. Robertson, C.T.R., authored a report (*Journal of Urology*, March 1992) comparing the perineal approach to surgery with the retropubic and found no substantial difference in time required, postoperative complications, or problems with positive surgical margins. They concluded that the perineal is an "excellent" approach and that which method is used depends on the preference and experience of the surgeon.

The other surgical approach is "retropubic." It is the most used. The retropubic method enters the patient in "the front," with an incision from the navel to the pubic bone, and allows access to the lymph nodes draining the pelvic areas. These nodes are removed and pathologically analyzed prior to proceeding with the surgery. However, many surgeons these days do not wait for the pathology results but go ahead with the radical prostatectomy. If the nodes turn out positive for cancer, they will proceed unless gross disease is found. This is not a universal concept, and other surgeons, upon finding tumor in the lymph nodes, will not proceed with the prostatectomy. We described the laparoscopic method of lymph node examination earlier.

Let Dr. Nash explain: "There are several views regarding the significance of tumor in the pelvic lymph nodes . . . the Mayo Clinic and other centers will go ahead with removal of the prostate even if a small amount of tumor is present, because in their opinion the data does show that if early endocrine ablation, that is, hormonal treatment or orchiectomy, is added at this time, the patients will have a prolonged time to recurrence if the tumor is diploid and the likelihood of extended survival is enhanced. This conclusion is not universally accepted."

In addition to the medical reasons for proceeding with surgery in all but gross disease discovery, surgeons do not want to have to tell a patient they "closed him up" without removing the prostate. They know this information sends the patient into deep concern, possibly depression. Whatever the physician tells him about potential relief from other treatment methods, the patient often feels his doom is sealed and begins to live in contemplation of pending death, whereas under treatment his death may be years in the future.

Reports as recent as 1991 support Dr. Nash's contention that the tumor-free survival percentages for a radical prostatectomy for early cancers—A1, A2, and B1—are 20 percent greater at fifteen years than similarly reported radiation therapy results. However, to qualify for this operation, you must have a life expectancy of ten years or more, pass a thorough cardiac evaluation, and be otherwise in good general health. Usually, the age cutoff is seventy, but the health of the patient may change that. One doctor quipped, "I'd never do a man as old as seventy-two unless his father brought him in to me."

The Operation

Your doctor will explain that the operation may leave you temporarily or permanently incontinent and temporarily or permanently impotent. Total incontinency occurs in less than 1 to 2 percent, and potency varies according to the patient's age and the extent of the tumor with less subsequent potency in older men. But potency sometimes may not return for as long as two years. There are ways you can be helped in the meantime. (See chap. 18 on potency.)

If medically qualified and aware of the possibility of complications, the patient will be delayed six to eight weeks, in some places as long as three months, to allow biopsy sites to heal. While waiting, he'll usually store up to three units of his own blood and will be given iron supplements so that at surgery he has a normal blood volume. During the operation the average blood replacement is two to three units although frequently no additional blood is administered. There are times when more is given. Preoperative hormonal treatments (Lupron) may shrink the prostate and contribute to less blood loss.

Dr. Walsh notes that at one time "profound blood loss" was encountered to the point that once major blood vessels were cut, the operation was completed "blindly and bluntly." The newer procedures prevent this problem and Dr. Walsh confirms that only 2 percent of his patients require additional transfusions in excess of their own stored blood. The advances also avoid a serious postoperative problem of possibly dangerous blood clots.

"Thus," he wrote, "radical prostatectomy can be performed today in a relatively bloodless, controlled fashion and is rarely associated with postoperative complications."

The night before the operation you will be given a cleansing enema, a liquid diet and, with some surgeons, a bowel prep in case there is any bowel injury, which occurs occasionally. Such injuries are usually repaired during the surgery and ordinarily do not require a diverting colostomy, although friends who enjoy forecasting dismal outcomes will "help" you with warnings of same. The anesthetic probably will be epidural (fluid dripped into the epidural space of the spine, the space around the spinal column) with or without a general anesthetic.[3]

Your legs will be wrapped and perhaps receive intermittent pressure to prevent swelling. This helps venous return and prevents pooling of the blood and possible blood clots. A specific description of each step of the procedure necessarily involves detailing numerous nerves, blood vessels, and tissues to be severed and repaired, and you can identify those when you go for your medical degree. I have a complete, detailed surgical description of a prostatectomy and, without a medical dictionary, identified primarily the prepositions, articles, and conjunctions. During the operation any blood lost is recycled, using a "cell saver," and can be reprocessed and transfused back into you during or after the operation.[4]

It is sufficient for our purposes here to say that your entire prostate and seminal vesicles will be removed, tissue preserved for later lab analysis, and, if possible, one or both of the neurovascular (nerves and blood vessels) bundles on either side of the prostate carefully separated from the capsule and left intact. Preserving even one of these may save your erection for when you feel better again. If your cancer is close to the bundles or is on both sides of the prostate too near the bundles for assured separation, one or both bundles will be sacrificed to get rid of the cancer.

A catheter will be inserted and a new bladder neck formed to be joined to the urethra by sutures. The bladder will be irritated to make sure the joining of these tubes, known medically as an *anastomosis*, is OK. This joining is infrequently a cause of postoperative problems but usually these are easily handled. A drain will be placed and the wound closed. If you had an epidural anesthetic, the catheter—a little short one you won't even know is there—will be left in place for several days to provide either a steady or intermittent drip, controlled by the anesthesiologist, to offset any pain while you heal, but you'll remain mentally alert while it is at work. Pain doesn't always occur, but the catheter is there in case it does. The operation will take from two and a half to three hours.

You'll go to an intensive care unit for one to three days so your immediate recuperation can be monitored. By the first night, certainly by the second day, they'll get you out of bed and gradually increase your walking around. You'll be fed, lightly, as bowel functions return, and you'll get some antibiotics during this time.

After four or five days, you'll be eating, passing some gas, and walking around, and six to ten days after the operation you'll go home. For a week or so, according to friends who've been through this drill, you'll move as though something hurts, because it will. After all, you have a sizable wound. In another week, you can be out and around but not jitterbugging or pressing iron because there'll still be a catheter draining out of your penis into a plastic bag strapped to your leg. About twenty-one days after the operation the urinary catheter will be removed, which process, to you, will surpass as a reward most other major events in your life, including graduation from high school.

A study of a large number of patients at Johns Hopkins showed that 50 percent of their patients regained urinary control at about three months. Many will take longer. Your control will return first at night, then during the day and finally you'll have control even when you cough or sneeze or fart. For a while, you will do any of these carefully.

About half regain urinary continence in about three months, 89 percent within a year, and 92 percent after two years, to cite a major recent study. No one in that study remained totally incontinent, but a few needed extra assistance, such as installation of a urinary sphincter. Meanwhile, ask about exercises that will strength your control. A drug, Ornade, may help.

Shortly after surgery, within four to six, perhaps eight, weeks, you will have a follow-up PSA test. If it is zero or near zero, you can relax. This means there is no residual, measurable cancer remaining. Infrequently, it may take as long as a year for the PSA to decline to the 0.1 to 0.3 "good news" level. It may hang around 0.2 for a while. These are Hybritech readings. Hybritech is one of several PSA assays. They are not precisely the same, so technically designation of the assay used is important. A borderline PSA is tough to analyze immediately, say 0.4 ng/ml. From that point it may decline over time. If it doesn't, even a small PSA elevation indicates all the tumor was not removed or there are distant metastases that weren't apparent before. An elevation in PSA likely will lead you to further treatments in time, either by radiation or hormonal blockade or both. Depending on the test, your doctor may wait and see or he may proceed with additional treatment right away. If he or the pathologist strongly suspect some tumor remains at the operation's margins or in your lymph nodes, you may receive hormonal treatment immediately or radiation in three months.

Prior to the operation, your doctor may have had reason to suspect a problem, and if so, he asked if you prefer hormonal drugs or an orchiectomy in case the disease turned out at surgery to be pathologically more extensive than it appeared clinically, before the surgery. Now, that's a decision you want to be prepared to assist in making. Again, there's disagreement about timing, but the weight of opinions leads toward starting hormonal therapy immediately if circumstances require the treatment.

Combined Treatments

With B3, C, and D stage cancers, a radical prostatectomy rarely is the original treatment of choice. Surgery in D1 clinically staged cancers is not usually recommended but happens when the cancer turns out to have been understaged or lymph node invasion is discovered either during the procedure or afterward by further examination in the pathology lab. Or perhaps the first node report might have been negative but a further study showed nodes positive. A study of a small series of operations that turned out be on D stage cancers showed some patients remained disease-free for eight years, which was the age of the study to that time. Another series of 64 patients treated with radical prostatectomy, but not hormonally, reported 70 percent disease-free at forty-eight months, with results scaling downward over the years. Dr. Nash points out that this is why the Mayo group recommends early hormonal blockade, at the time of surgery, in D1 stage cancers.

The American Cancer Society reported that only 1.1 percent of 23,000 men treated for prostate cancer in their survey in 1990 underwent radical prostatectomies for stage D cancers.

When there are recurrences or when it is known some tumor remains in lymph nodes, prostatectomies have been followed by radiation or radiation combined with androgen ablation (either hormones or orchiectomy).

Even in the case of D cancers this has met with moderate long-term success, especially when the tumor is diploid; not so much if it is aneuploid.

Following surgery, if any cancer has been discovered around the margins of the excised specimen, or extending beyond the capsule, postoperative radiation will be employed. Drs. Irving D. Kaplan and Malcolm A. Bagshaw, of Stanford University, and Dr. Jean deKernion, UCLA, in separate reports found that radiation begun three to four months after surgery, allowing time for healing, resulted in 90 percent of their patients remaining clinically free of disease for seven to nine years.

Disease evidence in organs or tissues removed at surgery may require postoperative radiation therapy or hormonal blockage; if in lymph nodes, hormonal blockage. Dr. Nash treats early those patients in whom he finds evidence of potential recurrence, i.e., capsular penetration, positive margins, involvement of seminal vesicles, especially if the tumor has a high Gleason grade, or in whom the PSA rises or does not fall. If the physician waits for clinical evidence of recurrence, either by palpation or biopsy, favorable results may be cut in half.

The Mayo clinic tracked 294 patients starting in 1970 on whom immediate orchiectomies were performed following radical prostatectomies in which lymph nodal disease was discovered. They reported disease-free survival in 80 percent at five years, 77 percent at 10 years, and 64 percent at 15 years, a rather high rate of success when compared to broader based survival records for D1 cancers. Mayo concluded that when hormonal treatment (orchiectomy, in this study) was delayed the results were not that good by half. Once again my reading confirmed that DNA ploidy is a significant factor in disease-free survival. In the Mayo series no patient with diploid tumors and early hormonal treatment following surgery had a recurrence of his cancer. Those who failed were not diploid.

Your doctor can tell you whether your cancer is diploid or aneuploid at any given biopsy if you want to know. He may tell you anyway if that is his policy, but he may also want to know whether you can handle what may be discouraging news.

For example, the Mayo people also reported that disease-free rates of survival in cases of limited nodal metastasis treated with surgery and followed by early hormonal ablation (orchiectomy) were better than in single treatment methods (monotherapies) except for patients with aneuploid—not diploid—tumors. Forty percent of the patients in this study with stage D disease had diploid tumors, and among them there has been no disease progression with the combined therapy.

Support for radical prostatectomies over other treatments for advanced cancers arose in a prepublication report from Duke University

Medical Center, Division of Urology, sent us courtesy of Dr. Paulson. It found that "patients with limited node positive disease selected for radical prostatectomy experience a survival advantage over those denied such therapy, and this is independent of adjunctive (additional therapy, such as hormonal or radiation) therapy." Drs. Frazier and Paulson, with C.T.R. Robertson, authored the report.

This is in conflict with other studies claiming that hormonal treatment upon discovery of lymph node invasion has established improved survival, but it also corroborates earlier random findings that prostatectomies on C and D1 cancers where nodal invasion was found contribute significantly to longevity in a high percentage of patients.

Dr. Frazier and his colleagues studied 156 patients treated between 1975 and 1989, all of whom were originally staged A or B but were found at pathology to have metastasis in lymph nodes. Some of these underwent radical prostatectomies and others did not have their prostates removed. Median survival for the removed group was 10.2 years and for the non-removed was 5.9 years. However, if three or more nodes were positive there was no difference in survival. Also, they found neither immediate hormonal treatment nor postoperative radiation improved survival.

Once again, the wisdom of regular examinations and early discovery shows through the statistics. The earlier the finding, the more likely it will be that diploid tumor cells predominate and the higher the cure rates will be.

Hormonal Treatment in Advance of Surgery

Another approach receiving attention in the United States and Canada is the potential of downstaging prostate cancer with "neo-adjuvant therapy," that is, either complete or partial hormonal blockade prior to radical surgery.[5]

Some cancer centers offer neo-adjuvant therapy to patients for three months before surgery. The doctors use Lupron or Zoladex combined with flutamide to check both testicular and adrenal testosterone. With B3 and C stage cancers, neo-adjuvant therapy may be used for six months rather than three.

They can't make a tumor go backward, that is, from a C to a B, for instance, but frequently they can shrink the size of the tumor, possibly making for an easier operation with the hope of lower blood loss. Yet there is always a qualification: some studies have claimed reducing a stage C cancer to a B2. Remarkable!

Although there is more preoperative use of hormonal therapies these days, there is a viewpoint that such treatments may improve the quality of a patient's life for a time but do not extend survival. On the other hand, some reports on combined surgery-hormonal therapy suggest any successes should be credited to the hormonal treatment, which might have done the job without the surgery.

What's an underinformed but deeply concerned layman supposed to think? Read Dr. Nash's counsel herein on how to select your professional mentors, and if satisfied with your choices, debate and then follow their philosophies. All in all, preoperative hormones may be like chicken soup for a bad cold: they might not help, but they couldn't hurt if they stop the cancer from growing for a few months.

15

Hormonal Ablation
Blocking Your Androgens with Surgery or Drugs

The relative absence of clinical endocrinologists specialized
in the endocrinology of prostate cancer can possibly explain the
important delay in the application of basic endocrine
knowledge to therapy of this disease.
FERNAND LABRIE, M.D., Ph.D., F.R.C.P. (C.)

WHEN YOU SHOW UP at your urologist's office and are examined for the first
time, physicians call this "presenting." They'll say, "this patient 'presented' with a lesion of about two cm in the prostate gland, a PSA of 5.2,"
etc. It's part of their reporting shorthand.

I've come across a variety of figures concerning the seriousness of
prostate cancers at patient presentation. Different reports say that from 30
to 70 percent of new prostate cancer patients "present" with disease that
has already escaped the prostate capsule. Around 30 percent show metastases in lymph nodes, other organs, or bone. This is serious stuff. It means
that in thousands of men cancer has been growing unnoticed for a long
time and has extended beyond curability (but still may be controlled). Recently, however, because of PSA-related earlier discovery, it does seem that
these adverse statistics are declining.

In such cases, or when the cancer recurs after previous therapy, the
principal treatment since the 1940s, has been hormonal. Prostate cancer is
especially reactive to male hormones, called androgens. Testosterone is
the male androgen, or hormone. Estrogen is the female hormone. Most
prostate cancer cells appear to depend on androgens for their growth.
Hormone-related treatment may also be important in female diseases related to the sex system, including certain types of breast or uterine cancer.

Thus with more advanced prostate cancers a major therapy consists of
removing the main testosterone source, the testicles. We have referred before to a surgical procedure called a "bilateral orchiectomy," which may
not require even an overnight stay at the hospital. It takes the testicles and a
substantial part of your testosterone away.

Major new studies strongly suggest that the sooner hormonal treatment begins, the better it works. Since we are talking about prostate cancer, you should know that equally convincing arguments maintain immediacy is not critical to survival.

There are drugs that have the same effect as the surgery: Lupron and Zoladex, for two. But you have to take them the rest of your life, by monthly injection. Even the monthly interval is only a few years old; previously, shots had to be given daily. Currently, Lupron runs about $500 to $600 a shot, Zoladex about $100 less. Prices vary and these aren't guaranteed. Cy Nash tells a patient, "I can take your testicles for about $3,000 (including hospital, anesthesia, etc.), or I can give you shots every month for about $6,000 a year. Which do you prefer?"

He's not surprised when the patient chooses the shots, as many do, although he says emphatically that if it were his problem he'd choose castration. For one thing, Medicare insurance frequently picks up the tab, so the cost doesn't bother most patients who have achieved Medicare status. For another, men, even older men, find surgical castration difficult to handle psychologically. It means a loss of sex drive (libido). So do the shots, of course. But deep in the recesses of his mind, the patient fears feeling less manly with his testicles gone. After all, he has protected the "family jewels" all his life and regarded them as evidence of his virility. You remember the old saw: "'Balls,' said the queen, 'If I had one I'd be king.'"

At this level of prostate cancer (recall, we are talking about advanced cancer, perhaps a C2 or C3, or a D1 or worse), the patient is in a life-threatening situation. Unless he is already well along in years, he may die of prostate cancer, rather than with it, as men with localized disease may more frequently expect. As far as potency is concerned, he may have to decide whether he wishes to attempt to prolong his life or to continue his sex life without a drug or mechanically assisted erection.

If his cancer has metastasized into bone, depending on how many bony lesions have developed, without treatment he could be facing death within eighteen months to two years, or sooner. There are exceptions: Cy Nash has had a few orchiectomized patients who've made it into their nineties, living ten years or more after diagnosis.

He told me, "If the man has pain in his bones, for instance, he's got a D2 cancer and he's in pretty bad shape. But we've had patients who have lived for ten years with a D2. I have a man now whose testicles I took off twelve years ago and he's living. He's still got cancer, but he's alive. So about 10 percent of patients with D2 bone cancer can go ten years or more and have a full life with proper hormonal treatment."

I asked if a man in that condition could function without some debilitation. His answer was yes. "We want an impact on survival. The real impact comes in catching it earlier. The cures are better if you get it early, no matter how you treat it." I had to comment that counting on being part of that 10 percent was still relying on fairly long odds.

The basic idea with extended disease is to deny the cancer its hormonal nourishment. A major shift in treatment occurred in the past ten years or so. Formerly, men with metastatic cancer were given diethylstilbestrol (DES), a synthetic estrogen or female hormone. In the seventies, a major research project in Veterans Administration hospitals confirmed that doses of DES slowed down, or reduced pain, in about 70 to 80 percent of advanced prostate cancer patients. The dosages started with 5 milligrams of DES daily. But DES also acts as a hyper-coagulant and causes fluid retention, contributing to heart problems.

It soon became evident that more patients were being lost to cardiovascular problems caused by the DES than to the prostate cancer. Doses were reduced to three mg, then to one. The small dose seemed to be about as effective as the larger one and sharply reduced the side effects of heart and circulatory disorders but didn't eliminate them altogether. Today, treatment with DES is not the norm, though medical reports tracking patients back ten years or more report its use. It was what they had then.[1] However, for some patients who can't afford Lupron, low dose estrogen may be prescribed even today, plus low dose aspirin.

To stop testicular androgens without surgical castration, the Federal Drug Administration has approved the two so-called LHRH agonists, leuprolide (trade name Lupron) and goserelin (trade name Zoladex). LHRH stands for "luteinizing-hormone-releasing hormone.""Agonist" means "fighter against." I'm going into all this detail because if you do develop prostate cancer you're going to run across the LHRH agonists either in your reading about the disease or in your own treatment.

For our lay purposes, you can interpret "luteinizing" almost as defining a catalytic action that instructs the pituitary gland to increase its production of "gonadatropin [sex organ related] hormones."[2] In other words, the pituitary tells the testicles, "Make more of that stuff." The agonists block this stimulation. They say, "Turn it off," and have the same effect as an orchiectomy and are not as likely as DES to aggravate such side effects as breast enlargement or heart problems.

They can present a short-term problem. They may temporarily cause a flare in tumor growth which recedes in less than two weeks. So their use in men already in pain may be limited unless the flare is checked by other medication. When this may be a concern, drugs called antiandrogens—"against" androgens—are administered before the agonists. Flutamide (trade name Eulexin) and nilutamide are antiandrogens.

Since Lupron or Zoladex block the body's ability to make use of testosterone they cause impotence. They may also give men that reportedly common symptom of menopause in women, hot flashes, for a similar reason: hormonal flow is interrupted. I was on Lupron for two months between my TURP and the start of radiation therapy and I experienced a few flashes. Not a serious affliction but you know when they hit. The flash is like stepping up close to a hot stove for a few seconds.

Although the testicles normally produce about 90 percent of your body's testosterone, your body doesn't quietly surrender to tinkering around with its hormonal supply system. With your testicles out of action, your adrenal glands, sitting there atop your kidneys, try to make up the loss and will produce directly and indirectly about 40 percent of your previous testosterone quantity, including small amounts from the skin and other bodily mechanisms, possibly the prostate itself if you still have one. To stop the uptake from these secondary sources, medicine turns to the direct antiandrogen drugs such as flutamide or nilutamide.

Combined with an LHRH agonist this treatment stops just about all testosterone use. Antiandrogens are also prescribed in combination with orchiectomy to cut off all hormonal nourishment to the cancer.[3]

Reporting on a large series of tests sponsored by the NCI at various cancer centers, Dr. E. David Crawford of Denver noted that a combination of flutamide and Lupron resulted in longer survival than Lupron or orchiectomy alone and delayed progression of the disease, especially in low volume cancers.

Three Canadian doctors, Fernand Labrie, Andre Dupont, and Alain Belanger, of the Laval University Hospital in Quebec, have been leaders in the study of combined LHRH agonists, or orchiectomy, plus flutamide treatment. Some other researchers feel they've been overenthusiastic in their reportage, but if all researchers agreed on every announcement in this field that would be more startling than Pasteur's basic discovery of germs.

In their original study (*Important Advances in Oncology*, 1991), Dr. Labrie and his colleagues applied complete hormonal treatment to more than 250 patients with stage C or D tumors. Of these, 84 had received no previous treatment. A group of D2 stage patients had been treated previously by castration or estrogens (DES). Their average age was sixty-seven, with a range from forty-eight to eighty years. They started the antiandrogen (flutamide) a day before the first administration of Lupron. Using both is known as "total androgen ablation," common enough now to be referred to in medical reports simply as TAA.

Substantial progress appeared in the previously untreated patients. Their PAP (prostatic acid phosphatase) dropped. Relief of pain came in a few days. Disease progression appeared to be halted. Changes were confirmed through digital rectal exams, transrectal ultrasonography, and other methods. All the previously untreated patients improved in appetite, sleep, and body weight and they "felt better." Improvements occurred in only 50 percent of those patients who had been previously treated with DES.

After a year, the Laval doctors' study showed far better results than earlier large-scale tests. The duration of response is critical, because although some patients on combined antiandrogen therapy have survived with the disease for several years, the majority have not.

Dr. Labrie and associates noted that their most important finding was that previously untreated prostate cancer, even at the late metastatic stage, "is exquisitively sensitive to androgens." Out of forty-seven patients who had the LHRH agonist or surgical castration plus flutamide, no disease progression was observed in anyone. Three cases relapsed after twenty-three months of treatment, and only one patient, described as terminally ill when treatment began, died after nine months, including six months of partial remission. Androgen deprivation treatment isn't new: what Labrie et al. added and asserted as confirmed was the effectiveness of the direct antiandrogen flutamide (there are others). They found that more than 99 percent of the tumors in stage D2 patients remained androgen-sensitive.[4]

Dr. Labrie says, "LHRH agonists should never be administered alone without the protection of simultaneous treatment with a pure antiandrogen" to prevent the flare syndrome and stop all androgen circulation.

In a later article, based on a talk Dr. Labrie gave at the National Conference on Prostate Cancer in San Francisco in February 1992, he called the combination therapy "imperative" as a first treatment where endocrine therapy is indicated because "monotherapy exposure shortens life by many months and those with a poor quality of life."

In tests the Labrie team conducted in Canada, the simple addition of flutamide to hormonal treatment was found to add 11.6 to 17.2 months of good quality life in cases of D2 cancer over and above the median two years, which is the best estimate, Dr. Labrie cites, of median survival achieved by orchiectomy, estrogens, or LHRH agonists alone. They mentioned also that in 5 to 10 percent of their patients, libido and erectile potency were maintained despite complete androgen blockade.

One critical difference rests with whether a patient has had previous treatment, with estrogens or orchiectomy, that blocked testicular testosterone only. Apparently, their earlier reports concluded, this "low level" or incomplete blockage allowed the development of "androgen-resistant" cancer cells, much as incomplete antibiotic treatment helps certain bacteria become resistant to antibiotics.

In more recent writings, Dr. Labrie sets aside the prevailing theory that some cells become insensitive to androgens. He urges now that belief be abandoned. Instead, he believes these cells are hypersensitive and can grow in the low androgen environment following orchiectomy. They thus require the extra further blockade of an antiandrogen.

What this adds up to, is that earlier hormonal treatment is better than later and that total blockade is essential in any case. On the other hand, by the early 90s there had not been total acceptance of the idea that orchiectomized patients should be treated forever with the flutamide combination. Dr. Labrie and his group strongly recommend that complete blockade be started as soon as possible after diagnosis of prostate cancer, especially those staged in the C and D categories, in order to improve survival. He now says emphatically that the negative effects of partial blockade or low androgen levels "make unethical the use of any therapy having lower androgen-blocking capacity than combination therapy." Strong language.

You can easily understand why Dr. Labrie's recommendations raised some medical eyebrows while at the same time stimulating additional research. Noting that there is a lifetime probability in the United States of diagnosis of prostate cancer in 5.6 percent of white males and 9.6 percent of black males, they assert that the "availability of a treatment that has no secondary effect, increases survival and permits resumption of normal activities with an excellent quality of life is of major importance." They recommend further that in all patients at stages C and D complete blockade should be initiated as first treatment, and that orchiectomy, estrogens, or LHRH agonists should no longer be used alone in this disease.[5]

When hormonal treatment doesn't work, cancer cells are said to be "hormone refractory." This is a nice way of saying, well, that hormonal treatment isn't working.

More studies are being analyzed of trials using flutamide and another antiandrogen, nilutamide. A February 1992 report in a way responded with understatement to the Labrie report saying that randomized trials in the United States and Europe have "shown a small but statistically relevant increase in progression free survival and even overall survival."

Hormonal blockade is being studied both in the United States and abroad for use in earlier cancers and even on localized cancers. Surgeons in several centers, when they find cancer in lymph nodes when operating or when lymph nodes are positive prior to surgery, put their patients on androgen ablation treatment; or, they may follow such surgery with radiation and sometimes combine androgen ablation and radiation. Not enough time has passed for specific analyses of these procedures.

Dr. Ralph W. deVere White, chairman of the University of California, Davis, Medical Center in Sacramento, stated in 1992 that neither monotherapy nor combination therapy is the answer to metastatic prostate cancer and that until we understand how hormones work we'll not truly be able to explain the therapies.[6] Nevertheless, Dr. White said, "there is hardly a single cancer study done where combination therapy, regardless of what it was, did not benefit the patients when compared with monotherapy."

Dr. White maintained that until something else becomes available, total androgen ablation should be "offered to patients with metastatic prostate cancer."

Early treatment also, theorized three Northwestern University Medical School doctors, could prevent or delay cancer cells from becoming aneuploid and could identify sooner patients who weren't responding and so permit a quicker start on other treatment methods. "The risk-benefit analysis . . . is strongly supportive of early hormonal therapy," they concluded. (More on this study in part 2.)

Our co-author Dr. Nash uses total androgen ablation on patients with advanced disease, employing either orchiectomy or Lupron for testicular hormone suppression. He and I spoke with several doctors attending a San Francisco conference in February 1992. They incorporated early and total blockade in their conversation as though there were no longer a question of its effectiveness.

They advocated aggressive, not conservative, treatment, for C and D stage cancers, especially D1's. The consensus seems clearly in favor of endocrine therapy as an adjuvant to radical prostatectomy (when that is possible in metastatic cases). They say that patients who had an orchiectomy at the time of prostate surgery live longer than those who delayed orchiectomy until progression of the disease if they had a stage D1, diploid cancer.

So our internal machinery clicks on. It probably was those burgeoning hormones that got us in trouble—or tried to—when we were teenagers, that determined our pursuit of sports, girls, and other standard enticements in our young adult years, and now, in our respective dotages, they are after us again. Now, however, we can readily suppress them, even if we do have to tell them goodbye with the deepest regret.

I think we might close this chapter with the anonymous quotation Drs.

Crawford and Nabors used to open their articles in *Urologic Clinics of North America* (vol. 18, no. 1, Feb. 1991):

"Then we have agreed that all the evidence isn't in and that, even if all the evidence were in, it still wouldn't be definitive . . ."

*   *   *

A little side note: between my early drafts of this chapter and the current rewrite, an interval of about eight months, the cost of Lupron rose to $546 a month. Flutamide treatment calls for six pills a day or about $360 per month. So we're talking about $10,000 a year for combined treatment. If the patient lives ten years on this regimen (not too likely), his cost goes to more than $100,000 if the price doesn't change. These drugs cost more if a hospital administers them. So, my prostate brother, if you are not on Medicare or you decide against losing your testicles, you have a problem . . . and so does your country's medical care budget. Dr. White said that if we were to take all patients diagnosed with metatastic disease over a three-year period and offer them either orchiectomy or LHRH agonists plus flutamide, the difference in expense to the country would be approximately $800 million a year. "It is thus extremely important that we understand just how hormonal therapy is working and identify the patients who will truly benefit from combination vs. monotherapy."

A recent study maintained that the cost of an orchiectomy compared to combined therapy was about even for the first two years. After that, the orchiectomy became much less expensive than the combination of drugs.

Advanced (C & D) Cancers
Serious Business, but Treatable

As prostate cancer advances, treatment strategies frequently change from those used on capsule-confined cancers. Let's hope a decreasing number of men will need the information herein.

A C STAGE PROSTATE CANCER (T3 by the international system), to save you looking it up, is localized to the prostate area but extends through the outer layer, perhaps into the seminal vesicles or the bladder outlet. A D indicates a tumor that appears to have, or has, extended beyond the prostate; a D1 has extended to the lymph nodes and a D2 indicates distant metastases, e.g., to the bones.

Treatment for stage C (clinical) prostate cancer opens another area if not of controversy then of dissatisfaction with the almost traditional avoidance of surgery in such cases. The medical journals indicate that more and more surgeons now attack stage C cancers with radical surgery and then add radiation or, increasingly, hormonal therapy.

Dr. Horst Zincke of the Mayo Clinic, noted that 44 percent of patients presenting with prostate cancer have clinical stage C disease. At surgery, many of those turn out to have been clinically overstaged and are pathological (that is, according to the pathology lab) B's; 42 percent are understaged and turn out to be really D1's. Only 36 percent in his ten-year study of 232 patients had confirmed stage C disease. Survival for these surgically treated patients, he said, "was significantly better than for a similar series of Stage C prostate cancer patients receiving radiation therapy alone."[1]

The whole gamut of therapies has been used on stage C prostate cancers: surgery, radiation, hormonal blockade, cryosurgery, implanted seeds (brachytherapy), and assorted combinations. How to treat this stage cancer, which is in a gray area between "localized" and "probably extended," frustrates doctors because reports of successes and failures range widely.

Dr. William H. Cooner, formerly of South Alabama College of Medicine and now at Emory University, Atlanta, says that if left untreated, half of clinical stage C patients develop metastases within five years. There will be a 23 percent recurrence in those irradiated. In one study, five-year survival was 69 percent; in another, 55 percent. A Stanford study reported that at five years 83 percent of their irradiated patients (348 patients followed for ten years) were free of local recurrence and at ten years, 36 percent. (Some had died of other causes.)

Dr. Zincke's ten-year study involved 232 stage C patients who underwent radical prostatectomies. He said their survival rates were significantly better than that of clinical C patients receiving radiation therapy alone. He also advocates, in selected cases, using adjuvant (along with) hormonal therapy to improve single-treatment methods.

Dr. Zincke and a Mayo team in a later published analysis reviewing more than a thousand men who had radical prostatectomies for pathological stage C cancers found 53 percent had unsuspected extracapsular extension.[2] Limited extension proved not more serious than organ-confined disease, but further extension or seminal vesicle invasion was "associated with a significantly poorer prognosis." Crude survival figures, meaning there may have been some cancer evident, for the men in the study were good, slightly better than would be expected in the population at large: 91 percent for five years; 68 for 10 years; and 46 percent at fifteen years.

The key points, the doctors concluded, were that postoperative treatment by either radiation or orchiectomy decreased disease progression but did not improve survival figures. Such treatment did, however, help control recurrences. Five-year recurrence-free experience for the treated men was greater than 95 percent, while for those not given adjuvant treatment it was 84 percent.

Very likely, we have seen in several reports, the biologic aggressiveness of the tumor measured by its grade and bulk will have more bearing on the patient's outcome than whether there is minor residual tumor remaining after a prostatectomy. The question of early added treatment following the operation is fraught with variables and conflicting ways of measuring and qualifying what is measured. The issue returns to the patient's condition, the biology of his cancer, and specific assessments of an individual's symptoms. Some centers think they should respond only to evidence of disease progression; some use follow-up radiation on all operations for C stage cancer. The hard fact is they all wind up with close to the same results, which are closely related to Gleason grade and ploidy status.

Your doctor may want to examine your lymph nodes. There is a greater chance that some cancer has escaped the prostate capsule with a C than with a B. One report claimed that with a PSA below 40 ng/ml there was only a small chance of lymph node invasion but there's ample disagreement with that, as well. PSA's of less than 15 strongly suggest no bone metastases are present. In clinical C's, about 60 percent of patients will have some lymph node tumor. You'll endure the standard range of tests and scans plus a prostatic acid phosphatase (PAP) blood serum test. The PAP is deemed useful in documenting metastases, if any. If you are headed for the linear accelerator and you have a urination problem, you may have a TURP (transurethral resection of the prostate) first. If you are headed for a radical prostatectomy, of course, the TURP is unnecessary.

The most commonly used therapy for clinical C's is radiation. The next most popular therapy is hormonal, followed by prostatectomy, which is seeing rapidly increasing application. Combined treatments are increasing, that is, prostatectomy followed shortly thereafter with either radiation (external beam) or hormones.[3] If Dr. Nash finds lymph nodes invaded, either during surgery or in examinations after surgery, his current course is to give hormonal blockade immediately.

There's discussion of whether hormonal treatment after surgery should be started immediately or delayed until some evidence of the disease reappears. The consensus seems to follow the Labrie dictum we reported in the chapter on endocrines—don't wait.

The facts are that given different ploidy analyses, some cells apparently resistant to radiation, and some cells apparently immune to hormonal blockade, your individual situation needs thorough study and candid discussions with your doctor(s). Variations on the treatment themes are being tried. For example, giving hormonal treatment before surgery to attempt to reduce the tumor burden and the size of the prostate to facilitate the surgery; or using newer techniques of transrectal ultrasound in guiding the placement of implanted radioactive seeds.

While it is true that medicos feel they have not yet solved stage C treatments to their satisfaction, the five- and ten-year survival and disease-free figures are encouraging to today's victims. They could be a lot worse.

There seems to be general agreement that DNA ploidy is a strong indicative factor in the probable success of treatment, with diploid a much more optimistic condition for the patient than aneuploid or tetraploid biologies.

Stage D Prostate Cancers

Stage D1 cancers—meaning lymph node invasion but not distant metastases—are complex, and the medical fraternity is as interested in improving the quality of life of these threatened patients as in prolonging their survival. Toward both these goals, surgery, radiation, and androgen ablation, including drugs and orchiectomies, have been pursued. Again, surgery together with hormonal ablation has become a more popular option in the 1990s.

Dr. David F. Paulson, professor and chief of urology at Duke University Medical Center, graciously sent us a prepublication copy of a study performed by Dr. Harold Frazier II, C.T.R. Judith E. Robertson, and himself. They found median survival rates for D1 patients who underwent radical prostatectomies double that for those who did not have their prostates removed: 11.2 years for those who did vs. 5.9 for those who did not. The entire cohort of patients in this study had prostate lymph node dissection, so the surgical and nonsurgical patients were well matched for this study.

Interestingly, in view of somewhat (but not exactly) similar studies, the Duke team found in the radical prostatectomy patients that the adjuvant treatment with immediate androgen deprivation or postoperative radiation did not improve survival; that removal of the prostate itself was the key factor in the survival difference. In the group not treated surgically (except for the lymph node dissection) they found a significant survival advantage with radiation therapy over those observed with no treatment, 6.5 years vs. 3.9 years.

Neither early or delayed hormonal deprivation provided a survival advantage among the patients who did not have a radical prostatectomy.

This crisply written report defies easy condensation, so these are the highlights. Patients with one or two positive lymph nodes had 10.2 years cancer-specific survival if a prostatectomy was performed but 5.9 years if not; patients with three or more positive nodes did not benefit from radical surgery. The report hypothesized that "surgical debulking of malignant and benign prostatic tissue may deprive remaining malignant tissue of endogenous [influenced by other elements within the body] growth factors." In other words, removal of the prostate may have removed the principal source of tumor and much of whatever was stimulating its spread.

In another report almost at the same time, a group from the Mayo Clinic and Mayo Foundation found that D1 surgical patients who had DNA diploid cancers and received early endocrine therapy did significantly better than a similar group that did not have immediate endocrine treatment.[4] Nondiploid patients received some disease-free survival benefit with early endocrine therapy but no benefit in terms of delayed death from their cancers.

Reports from the Mayo Clinic seem to be highly collegial. Another published in July 1992 in a *Cancer* supplement (vol. 70, no. 1), led by Dr. Horst Zincke with several members of the team that produced the above research, found evidence for favorable survival in surgical patients given immediate hormonal blockade treatment if their cancers were diploid. They estimated that only 20 percent of adjuvant hormone treated patients are likely to die within ten years. Diploid patients are unlikely to die in 10 years or less.

This also is a specifically categorized study with several qualifications to its conclusions that we needn't go into for our personal treatment decisions. But the marked difference between the Duke report and the Mayo reports does show us the difficulty urology has in improving the enjoyable life span of D1 patients.

For men with D2 cancers, androgen deprivation by orchiectomy (removal of testicles) and antiandrogens, or Lupron or Zoladex plus the antiandrogen flutamide will be used. Trials using various chemical therapies are underway, but few specific reports are available because, unfortunately, results have been neither very good nor uniform, except for alleviation of pain. On the other hand, for about 20 percent of men with this advanced a cancer, total testosterone deprivation one way or the other has resulted in long-term survival.

It's your decision and your doctor will have some options that you might decide to try as opposed to doing nothing or simply relieving symptoms. Radiation, radical prostatectomy, chemotherapy have worked in some cases. Your individual situation and general health will be important in these decisions and your good cheer and fighting spirit may be even more important. I seem to be bogged down in all this clinical stuff, primarily because I'm dealing with medical information most patients rarely receive, but the state of your personal spirit is important not only psychologically but physically in helping your body battle this intruder.

I strongly recommend the late Norman Cousin's books on this topic: *Anatomy of an Illness* (Bantam Books, N.Y.), and *Head First* (Penguin Books, N.Y.). His explorations into the power of the mind in healing the body were so persuasive that he served as an adjunct professor of medicine at UCLA and received an honorary M.D. degree at Yale.

Recurrent and Residual Cancers
What If It Comes Back on Me?

**"Heard you had a cancer. How you doing?" "OK, so far.
Check me again in ten years."**

SORRY, BROTHERS OF THE PROSTATE, your initial treatment, be it radiation or surgery, may not "take." Those in the fraternity know it's difficult to answer the question from well-meaning friends, "I heard you had cancer. You look great. Are you cured?"

What do you say, "I'll tell you in ten years"? We know the prostate cancer can return. It can show up as a metastasis in some other part of the body. It may or may not come back as a localized cancer if it was localized at initial treatment. Or, fortunately for the majority of us, it may be gone for the rest of our lives. The point is, if we had a radical prostatectomy and survive ten years we are probably "cured." If we had radiation treatment and are now ten years older, say in our late seventies or mid-eighties, we still don't know for sure, though we may be at an age where we wouldn't care.

The new cryosurgical procedure hasn't been around long enough to analyze its long-term effectiveness as a primary or salvage procedure following radiation failure, but early trials raised hopes. With this process, if a tumor appears to still be in place six months or so after the first freeze treatment they can frostbite your prostate again. Newer techniques in this therapy are encouraging.

We're dealing with some picky definitions here. The reappearance of tumor might be a "recurrence" or "residual." *Residual* cancer is tumor tissue, perhaps microscopic, remaining after a surgical cure has been attempted. It might be found in the margins of the removed specimen or may have lingered in the lymph nodes. If positive nodes were found, the docs would assume there are probably more positive nodes extended in the lymph system chain. Residual cancer after radiation results in a positive biopsy eighteen months or so after treatment or in a rising PSA level after an earlier return to normal.

Recurrent cancer is one that appears at some time after initial treatment, perhaps even years later. Following radiation treatment, after the PSA has been down for a time, if the PSA begins to rise again and a biopsy shows cancer, your tumor has recurred. Whether something should be done about it and just what that would be, could keep a urologic conference debating for a weekend, with no time for golf or tennis.

Reappearances of prostate cancer generally are deemed "recurrences," although it is possible that a brand new tumor may have developed after the first was blasted with radiation. Perhaps radiation either didn't "get" all the cancer cells or merely stunned them for a long time. Perhaps some developed immunity to the rays. Or maybe there was unsuspected tumor in those unexplored lymph nodes. Increasingly deeper study of the significance of PSA changes holds that treatment will be needed if the PSA doubles in four months. (See chap. 26, part 2, on the PSA.)

Perhaps surgery, especially if the cancer was clinically understaged, left some cells at the margin of the prostate removal. Technically, the reappearance of cancer from microscopic cells remaining after surgery would be deemed "residual" rather than a recurrence, if you care what they call it. Perhaps there were distant but undetected cells that had migrated elsewhere and decided, after some months or years, to reassert themselves.

Unquestionably, the battle is turning toward the good guys. If your cancer is an A or B stage (confined to the capsule) at the pathological review of your operation you've a 95 percent chance of never hearing about it again, with a life expectancy as though you never had the disease at all. Whereas a few years ago upward of 40 to 50 percent of cancers turned out at surgery to be confined, more recently 70 percent are, indeed, confined as staged prior to your operation. This indication of progress reflects both improvements in staging methods and the fact that more cancers are being discovered early. Earlier discoveries mean more cancers can be cured. Finding the cancer early gives it less time to grow beyond the prostate.

If, at discovery of your cancer, your PSA is greater than 10, there's a two-thirds chance it has escaped the capsule. If greater than 20, there's a possibility it has spread to your lymph nodes. If your PSA is less than 10, there's a strong possibility it is still confined. Medicine makes every attempt to learn before treatment whether any tumor has extended beyond the capsule with biopsies, endorectal MRI coil scans, and so forth. There is no 100 percent certain process. After these exams, if there is extension, you probably would not have surgery.

My "coach" and co-author, Dr. Nash, if he finds omens of possible future recurrences, will give combined treatment at the outset, using radiation prophylactically (preventively) as soon after surgery as practicable if lymph nodes show no tumor. If nodes are positive, he would turn to hormonal blockade. Otherwise, following surgery urologists will routinely track PSA readings for indications that tumor has invaded the margins of the operation. Or an undiscovered invasion of lymph nodes may show up in the lab examining the surgical specimens. We are now into a situation so dependent on individual diagnostic circumstances I hesitate to generalize, but, in general, local extension (especially in high Gleason grades) would call for radiation follow-up, and distant extension for hormonal therapy.

Every effort will be made before a radical prostatectomy to determine whether there is tumor outside the gland: biopsies of the seminal vesicles and of the neurovascular bundles, MRI exams of the seminal vesicles, endorectal MRI, transrectal ultrasound visualization of the capsule, PAP tests—all to learn if a surgical attack can be avoided on what might be discovered, under the microscope of the pathology lab, to be a stage C tumor. Again, none of these tests yields perfect answers.

The largest group of recurring cancers appears in men who were clinically understaged prior to their operations and were found at pathological assessment to have seminal vesicle invasion, other tumor outside the capsule, and/or "positive margins" of the surgery, that is, cancer at the very edges of the removed tissue (meaning that it might be in the very edges of the remaining tissue, too). Rather than wait for a recurrence to appear, most urologists suspecting a chance of future trouble would treat with radiation three or four months after the surgery.

In cases of surgery done despite the finding of cancer cells in lymph nodes as the operation began, hormonal therapy in addition (adjuvant) to the original surgery may delay or even prevent recurrence. Whatever the cause, prostate cancers do recur. This is why patients are followed regularly by their doctors, given periodical PSA and PAP tests, and biopsied if these are elevated following original treatment.

Wait! Diversion coming! My wife and over-the-shoulder editor says this is too grim and scary. Perhaps I've gotten into this subject too deeply and am becoming desensitized. Statistically, if you have a capsule-contained tumor and a capable surgeon you have a 95 percent chance of total cure, no recurrence. Usually, radiation would address a more threatening tumor or one in an older man, not always. The better news is that although such recurrences produce elevated PSA's, even positive biopsies, frequently they may never threaten your general health. There are several reports of patients ten years after radiation therapy with elevated PSA's and no clinical evidence of cancer. There are similar reports of large numbers of postirradiation residual cancers evidenced by positive biopsies that showed no clinical evidence of disease progression over long time spans.

On average, radiation patients are seventy-three years old and after ten years will be eighty-three years old. A lot of us may not live that long, recurrence or not. With pacemakers, better cardiac care, and medical improvements across the board, many will live a lot longer than that, so don't stop your examination routine. A substantial number of cancers do recur.

OK, back to the grim.

Whether the cancer reappears, when evidence of reappearance is discovered, the stage and grade of the original tumor and the recurring one, and whether the original treatment was by surgery or radiation may bear on how to deal with its return. If it comes back on you, whether the cancer was subjected to hormonal blockade prior to its reappearance would affect the decision as to subsequent treatment. Breaking down each conceivable category of possible problems and assigning a possible treatment to each would make your eyes glaze over by the second paragraph.

But the possibility is why, once treated by any mode, you will be examined regularly and monitored carefully just in case. Moreover, procedures have changed so much in the last ten years that even the statistical gurus who keep up with the variations caution readers that their figures are general guides and not as specific, for instance, as your average number of income tax returns filed. What they're saying is that if some therapy didn't work well ten years ago improvements in techniques may have it working better today.

If after radiation the PSA count drops to a low level, even below 1.0 ng/ml, and then begins to rise again you'll want additional tests every six months, perhaps every three. The rate of the rise will be significant. If the count exceeds 4.0 ng/ml you'll probably encounter a series of tests to determine whether further treatment will be necessary. A positive biopsy eighteen months or later or a rising PSA, or both, would define a residual cancer.

Dr. Paul F. Schellhammer and colleagues at Eastern Virginia Medical School raised several questions about failures after radiation, even of definition and of what is really meant by "failure."[1]

That's a good question with no one definitive answer. It means the first procedure did not achieve an absolute cure. In some patients failure might mean a positive biopsy; in others an elevated PSA. In some circumstances signs of failure might lead merely to further testing of items like PSA doubling time (see chap. 26 in part 2). Appearance of metastasis signaled by pain means failure.

First indications of failure probably will show up at one of your periodic PSA tests. As a "graduate" of earlier treatment you will be tested regularly, at three, six, and twelve months, and then at least once a year for all time. If you show an elevation in your PSA, even a small one, your doctor will schedule subsequent tests maybe three or four months apart. The time between an early test and next test, or the ones after that, strongly suggests the time it will take for the failure to manifest itself sufficiently to be so labeled. The rate of change in PSA is significant, underscoring the need to take your post-initial-treatment exams on time.

Whether the cancer is well or poorly differentiated will affect determination of the recurrence's significance. Your doctor will want to know just what he is dealing with and the same assessments confronted when your cancer first appeared will have to be repeated. In a younger person with a rising PSA treatment is called for; slow doubling time in an older patient could mean no further treatment.

The Eastern Virginia team noted that though failure may not manifest itself for five or ten years, most radiation patients eventually will fail. However, after eleven years of follow-up in their studies, four of twenty-two biopsy positive patients are still absent any clinical evidence of disease, indicating that their cancers weren't killed outright but were stunned into dormancy. So, it is possible to have biopsy-detected failure without serious disease progression.

Reporting on a minimum five-year follow-up with interstitially (implants) treated patients (iodine-125), Dr. Schellhammer et al. found no significant failures with stage A2 and B1 patients, 32 percent with B2 patients, and 44 percent with C patients. They found a 15 percent failure rate with patients with well-differentiated tumors, 36 percent with moderately differentiated tumors, and 54 percent with poorly differentiated tumors. It should be noted that these implants preceded the development of more accurate implant aiming techniques. We'll have to wait a few years to see how the newer procedures score. Doctors stopped using the older methods because of failures. Now they don't treat bulky tumors or stage C tumors with seeds. With stage B2 they may treat with external beam radiation first and add seeds later for more concentrated zaps.

These figures were not as good for B2 and C staged tumors as the figures for external radiation and surgical results. There's a statistical fallacy here, too, as older seeds methods can't be compared accurately with newer methods or with current methods of external beam radiation.

With that in mind, generally summarizing their collection of figures and charts, there were, as you'd expect, more failures with either radiation procedure than with surgery except for stage C surgery patients who, at both five- and ten-year levels, suffered more failures than radiation patients. The doctors reported that most researchers found a higher failure rate among patients with seminal vesicle involvement, and by now earlier dissidents to this view concur.

But statistics don't tell us much as individual patients, distressed that the treatment we've already endured didn't fix us permanently. Our question is, what are they going to do for us now that our PSA's are rising or it becomes otherwise clear that the cancer is gaining on us?

To thwart a returning cancer after radiation treatment, three "salvage" procedures top the menu: (1) surgery, under very special circumstances; (2) hormonal blockade with drugs or orchiectomy plus flutamide; (3) cryosurgery, which aims at freezing that sucker into oblivion. In extremely rare instances, practically unheard of, a second round of radiation might be used. Most doctors would not consider it.

In a paper presented before the American Urological Association 1994 annual meeting in San Francisco, Dr. Andrew C. von Eschenbach reported, "With over one year of experience with cryoablation [freezing] of the prostate, our data suggest that this is an ideal method of treatment for patients with local recurrence of tumor following definitive radiation therapy. The cryoablation has been well tolerated and over two-thirds have initially been rendered biopsy-negative in spite of the fact that recurrent tumors were of advanced stage and grade. We have recently modified our freezing technique in an effort to further enhance tumor cell destruction."[2]

Dr. von Eschenbach and his associates in this report are with the University of Texas M. D. Anderson Center in Houston, Tex. So far, they have used cryoablation only for the treatment of recurrent cancers following failure of radiation therapy, not as an initial treatment. (See earlier chapter on cryosurgery.)

Dr. Malcolm A. Bagshaw of the Stanford University Medical Center, a pioneer in the use of the linear accelerator in cancer treatment, remarked—and so have others—that if a tumor was not considered resectable (operable) before radiation, "it is unlikely to become resectable [by virtue of] radiation treatment."[3] Other experts' opinion as to radical surgery as salvage for failed radiation treatment range from "never" to "a procedure of desperation" because of percentages of aftereffects of incontinence and other problems. Nevertheless, some have produced good results.

Conditions for such surgery occur infrequently, Dr. Bagshaw wrote, but he said it is possible with careful selection and with "full appreciation of the increased risk for tissue injury due to reduced tissue tolerance." He reported a 50 percent disease-free survival rate for the procedure in his study. We don't know the details of the subset of patients who fared well with this treatment.

Dr. Bagshaw wrote that a positive biopsy without elevation of the PSA may mean the tumor cells are dormant, but that this is "clearly a troublesome circumstance and, unfortunately, one which has no clear resolution."

Drs. Judd D. Moul and David F. Paulson of the Duke University Medical Center, North Carolina, said the main issues are whether these operations can be done safely with acceptable morbidity (side or after-effects) and whether they prolong survival.[4] Drs. Moul and Paulson considered "failure" of irradiated patients to be a documented local or distant recurrence or a PSA elevated to more than 4.0 ng/ml.

Radical or extensive surgery to correct radiation failure, in other reports I read, resulted in unacceptable side effects to 25 percent of patients in one report, ranging up to 50 percent in others.

This figure was similar to that used by Dr. William Catalona in an editorial in the March 1992 *Journal of Urology* in which he questioned the increasing use of aggressive surgery. He does not recommend surgery for those who have failed radiation (nor for C and D stage cancers' initial treatment) claiming only 15 to 20 percent will have satisfactory outcomes.

Dr. Catalona finds no convincing evidence that the benefits of "radical surgery offset the associated risks in patients with advanced prostate cancer or in those who have failed radiation therapy. The available evidence suggests that hormonal therapy alone provides equivalent therapeutic benefits with less potential for morbidity."

So the disagreements continue among scientists in this field. Drs. Moul and Paulson found successes with salvage surgery, with good survival ratios. They believe that salvage surgery for "small volume recurrence . . . can be done without excessive morbidity and with reasonable disease control . . . in properly selected patients."

Advocates of surgery following failure of radiation say salvage prostatectomy might be tried on patients with a PSA of 10 or less who initially had a B1 or B2 carcinoma that appeared to be locally confined. One report said that 33 percent of such patients were helped, 50 percent had incontinence, and 15 percent some rectal involvement. But if it worked perfectly every time this would be an easy decision. As it is, if 50 percent fail it means 50 percent succeeded. Beats total failure, especially for the winners. Selection of patients for the procedure is a major item in success.

Should its apparent early successes continue, especially as skills and knowledge improve, cryoablation (freezing) could well turn out to be the weapon of choice in battling localized Sons of Cancer One. Dr. Nash's comments return us to the objective of all this discussion: we are not just fighting cancer in the abstract, we are fighting against the death of people.

The reappearance of cancer following a radical prostatectomy reawakens all those questions of defining the original tumor(s): grade, stage, patient condition, lymph node invasion, etc. Given a moderately accurate estimate of the cancer prior to surgery, your doctors first will try to prevent a recurrence or a reawakening of residual tumor cells remaining in the margins of an operation. With smaller tumors (A's and B's), unless these turn out at surgery to have been understaged, they'd expect first procedure success.

It is with C and D tumors (the latter are infrequently excised) that controversy arises. Should there be immediate added treatment or should it be delayed to see if problems emerge? Should the treatment be radiation or hormonal blockade? What are the patient's wishes? If the patient had a nerve-sparing operation, follow-up radiation will most likely thwart his desire for a return of potency, as would total androgen ablation. In such a case, depending on the extent of the tumor, a doctor might just wait and delay a second treatment. If your doctor thinks there may be some tumor left in the margins of your operation he'll probably tell you in advance that he will irradiate you as soon as possible postoperatively or start androgen ablation.

I have scattered across my desk, as I write, a dozen letters and articles by well-known physicians in the field. They are thoughtful and interesting, but they reflect a variety of views, some in strong conflict with each other.

Dr. Donald G. Skinner, of the University of Southern California School of Medicine at Los Angeles, found that patients with pathologic stage C lesions fared well with postoperative radiation, and concluded that his data supported a role for the treatment. Patients with high Gleason grades (8–10) and seminal vesicle involvement fared worst. Others experienced a minimum of problems from the radiation. Dosage was somewhat less than that used in an initial radiation course. Overall five- and ten-year survival was 94 percent and 70 percent respectively, and the chance of clinical recurrence was estimated at 6 percent and 13 percent. Dr. Skinner interpreted the study as supportive of a place for adjuvant radiation therapy following a radical prostatectomy.

Drs. Irving D. Kaplan and Malcolm A. Bagshaw of Stanford University,[5] and other researchers in separate studies, show results from excellent to poor in treating failed radical prostatectomy patients with radiation. Success may be affected by hormonal treatment prior to the radiation or by whether the recurring cancer is feelable in a DRE. A great deal, again, depends on your age, the staging of your original tumor, and the as-yet-unknown and frequently unreadable biological aggressiveness of the tumor itself, but Gleason grade and ploidy are important.

To summarize the Bagshaw-Kaplan findings, perhaps with only slight inaccuracy, some studies reported that postprostatectomy recurring patients had a better survival rate if they underwent radiation as a corrective procedure. The median age of the patients in their basic study was in the mid-sixties. Aftereffects of the treatment occurred in very few patients. These problems included swelling of legs and urethral strictures, but all were managed without complex treatment.

A team from the Palo Alto Medical Center and UCLA compared patients with local extension beyond the prostate gland and/or positive surgical margins who had added radiation with those who did not.[6] After ten years those with the radiation therapy registered 94 percent local control of their cancers and those treated with surgery alone showed 69 percent local control, a significant difference. Any impact on survival was not clear in this study.

Still, the benefits of postoperative radiation vary and when tumor is discovered in the margins of the former site of the now removed prostate (margin positive) there may be no survival difference between those who do and do not receive radiation. However, there may be a difference in quality of life.

A report from another UCLA group reviewed 115 patients who between 1976 and 1989 had radical prostatectomies for pathological stage C cancers and were at risk of progression. PSA tests indicated residual disease. Twenty-four patients had adjuvant radiotherapy and ninety-one did not. Eight patients died in the course of time: four in each group. Three of the four patients who had only surgery died of metastatic cancer and one of another cause. Of the radiation patients, one died of metastatic cancer and three of other causes. None of the twenty survivors who had radiation showed any clinical progression, but 25 percent showed PSA evidence of recurrence at five years and 46 percent at seven years. Clinical disease-free survival was 92 percent at five and seven years while the same figure for the surgery-only group was 67 percent at five years and 56 percent at seven. This report was briefed in the *Yearbook of Urology 1993* and the co-editor, Dr. J. Y. Gillenwater, commented that patients with local extension only should benefit from adjuvant radiation. Dr. Gillenwater noted that he uses adjuvant radiation for positive surgical margins and for patients whose PSA values do not fall to normal or become elevated.[7]

Dr. Nash thinks that any suspicion or pathological evidence of tumor in the margins of an operation calls for immediate follow-up radiation therapy. "Irradiate before it can establish itself; start early to prevent its return. We can often predict which ones are likely to return and treat before they do," he advises.

Dr. David F. Paulson of the Duke University Medical Center, who conducts and writes studies of markedly lucid detail and specificity, also concluded that immediate or early androgen deprivation provides no survival advantage in margin-positive recurrences although the treatments did delay evidences of progression.[8] Dr. Paulson's meaning is clear but the layman doesn't have to be a rocket scientist to see from the pivotal reports we've reviewed that postoperative therapy, hormonal or radiation, continues to be a seriously debated subject in the field.

With stage D1 patients, the trend is toward complete hormone therapy applied immediately following an operation. Indeed, this is frequently an initial treatment, accomplished by orchiectomy and drugs or drugs alone. In both C1 and D1 recurrences, hormone therapy has been fairly effective. Several small studies reported slightly higher than 50 percent prevention of further local growth or complications. A 50–50 chance isn't exactly heartwarming, but considering how advanced a D1 cancer is before treatment, it beats the alternative.

Dr. Horst Zincke of the Mayo Clinic, referring to cancers identified in the pathology lab as stage C, wrote that with older patients who show a rising PSA level, hormonal treatment will be used. Radiation is used with younger patients to retain their libido. He thinks that radiation will not improve survival, but that longer survival is possible in a subgroup of patients who have diploid tumors, and these will receive early hormonal treatment. His estimate of the situation depends more on rising PSA levels than on positive margins of surgery, as "positive margins may not be consistent with residual cancer."[9]

Dr. Jean B. deKernion, professor and chief of the division of urology at UCLA, advises radiotherapy only if there is extensive extracapsular extension. If there is microscopic nodal tumor he feels the risk is of metastases at distant sites and radiotherapy would be of little value. Postoperative patients, he says, are followed carefully, and if the PSA rises and follow-up biopsies are positive he would irradiate. If follow-up biopsies are negative, hormonal blockage would be the therapy of choice, depending on patient preference, age, and sexual function.[10]

I admire the explicit philosophy of Dr. William R. Fair, chief of urologic surgery at the Memorial Sloan-Kettering Cancer Center in New York. He wrote:

> I do not hold with those who feel that we should extend the indications for radical prostatectomy with the idea that if surgery fails we

can always give radiation to effect a cure. I find it is intellectually un-
satisfying to assume that radiation therapy is good treatment for prostatic cancer left behind after surgical treatment . . . and yet it is
inappropriate as primary treatment. . . . I do not believe that a surgeon should plan to do a radical prostatectomy on any patient except
those in whom he fully expects the surgery will remove all the
tumor. . . . We have no data that a combination of surgery and radiation is any more successful than radiation alone on controlling the
tumor or increasing longevity.

Dr. Fair would give postoperative radiation only to patients with a documented history of local recurrence. He's more inclined toward hormonal
therapy since it is systemic treatment and, at least theoretically, might benefit the patient no matter where the bad cells are located and might show a
survival advantage.[11]

Patients treated hormonally in addition to their initial treatment may
have a lower incidence of failure and take a longer time to fail, some studies
assert. Stages of cancers change. Ploidy of cancers change. Cell differentiation changes. Older studies can't be compared with fresher ones. Radical prostatectomies may have been retropubic or perineal (though with
newer techniques this shouldn't make a difference); lymph nodes may or
may not have been analyzed pathologically. If they have, the ploidy will be a
prognostic factor. We have better luck with diploid cancers. All these factors affect interpretation of statistics.

In addition to the question of what to do, there is a question of when to
do it. If the added treatment is to be hormonal, the general opinion seems
to favor starting immediately upon indication it may be needed. Some con-
tend with cancers discovered to be stage C or D pathologically, there are
significant survival benefits in avoiding delay. Their conclusion was that
immediate treatment, radiation or hormonal, decreased local and systemic
progression significantly but did not improve survival and that the issue
needs more targeted study.[12]

A victim's conclusion: added treatments will make us feel better
longer, but it looks as though the curtain will come down when the tumor
decides to ring it down regardless, if we have a C stage cancer and an elevated Gleason grade.

According to the American Cancer Society, about six thousand radical
prostatectomies were performed in the United States in 1988 and twenty-
three thousand in 1990, which testifies both to the growing popularity of
the procedure and improvements in discovery, but also demonstrates the
increasing difficulty of tracking how all those came out. Check again for

ten-year readings on prostatectomy failures in the year 2000. With screening and the PSA test more cancers are being discovered earlier, and so treatment should produce better survival and fewer recurrence figures.

By now, it is fairly obvious to the endangered layman that with a local recurrence he may face a true Hobson's choice: either undergo the unpleasant experience of extended and expensive medical attention—i.e., radiation after surgery, salvage surgery after radiation, or cryoablation after radiation—with the hope that life with some degree of quality can be extended several months to several years; accept total androgen ablation with the same hope; or wait to see what the cancer decides to do and battle the symptoms when they appear. Many doctors may not approve that last option. We are brought back to our often repeated phrase: it depends on the circumstances.

So, those of us who face a second course of treatment must resume our studies and probe our advisors deeply as to what procedures fit our problem and what the consequences of any treatment, as well as "no treatment," might be.

*   *   *

Please refer to Dr. Nash's counsel in part 2 about selecting your physicians. While he is discussing primarily your choice before diagnosis and original treatment, the rules apply to the doctors who will give you treatment if your cancer comes back. Some of the procedures mentioned in this chapter are not commonly practiced by every urologist. Dr. Bagshaw noted that surgery as a salvage procedure after radiation requires someone experienced in operating on irradiated tissues. Radiation as a adjuvant procedure after surgery should be under the control of especially qualified and experienced radiation specialists. It may appear that hormonal treatment consists merely of a shot once a month and a few pills every day, but proper dosages and trained awareness of your reactions to the drugs can be very important to your health. With the newer therapies such as cryoablation you don't have to play guinea pig while a doctor learns the techniques. Most of the failures of particular treatments might be written off as victories of the cancer cell over the treatment or over our slowly eroding ignorance of cellular behavior. But it is safe to assume that at least a few failures reflect insufficient skill and knowledge on the part of the practitioner concerning a procedure that may be beyond his experience or talents.

18

Potency
Will I Ever Get It Up Again?

**These days, any man can regain the ability
to have rigid erections, depending on how much
hassle he is willing to endure.**
LESLIE R. SCHOVER, PH.D.,

MOST MEN OLD ENOUGH to confront prostate cancer may not know much about the anatomy and mechanics of their erections, but unless they've been living in a monastery since puberty they do know that successful sex depends not on the mechanisms alone. Mental attitudes, emotional status, including the impact of being told you have cancer, plus the degree of patient and willing cooperation of one's partner bear heavily on potency.

Treatment for prostate cancer can affect your desire for sex, your ability to be sexually aroused, and your erection. It's not so much what happens to the prostate itself; to function sexually you could get along without one. Damage to your erectile ability depends on your treatment. External beam radiation may affect blood flow; unless a nerve-sparing technique is successful, both nerve–blood vessel complexes alongside the prostate could be lost or damaged in surgery; hormonal therapy blocks production of testosterone, the male hormone, and can reduce your desire as well as your ability. On the other hand, not to be vulgar about it, some studs aren't negatively affected by anything, given enough recovery time, desire, and stimulation.

Various ducts and glands associated with your ability to father children may be removed with surgery, but your erection may return in time and may do so after radiation, as well, depending on your potency prior to treatment and your age. Radioactive implants should leave you about the same as your pretreatment condition in this regard. There's been too little follow-through on the effects of the newer "freezing" procedures to comment knowledgeably.

The seminal vesicles provide a substantial portion of seminal fluid. In radical prostatectomies the seminal vesicles and the ducts that empty into the prostate will be removed along with the prostate. External beam radiotherapy will reduce or eliminate their function.

Our Virginia friend mentioned in the surgery chapter wasn't completely satisfied after one year with the return of his preoperation potency. He was using a vacuum device for augmentation. This is a plastic tube that fits over the penis. An attached hand pump creates a vacuum drawing blood into the penis and producing an erection. He complained to his urologist. The doctor told him to be patient a little while longer. "Part of your problem is psychological," he said. "You are worried about trouble and you are having a little trouble. Part of your problem is that you are seventy-two years old."

Studies of the role sexual activity may play in prostate cancer pretty well prove no specific causal relationship. Frequency of ejaculation, for example, seems to have no bearing on a tendency toward prostate cancer. Other studies that hinted that diminished sexual activity might cause trouble have not proved out over time.

A Japanese study that found that men with prostate cancer were less likely to have a history of sexually transmitted infections, had fewer premarital partners, and had less contact with prostitutes when matched against a group with benign prostatic hyperplasia. Data examining whether frequency of ejaculation might be linked to prostate cancer could be interpreted either way. Perhaps increased testosterone is a factor and perhaps sexual activity stimulates more testosterone, hypothesized some researchers. This theory didn't prove out, either. No such relationship was found and no excess generation of testosterone was determined.

Black Americans appear to develop prostate cancer earlier than whites. Their bodies generate about 15 percent more testosterone on average than whites. If this phenomenon has anything to do with the higher rates of affliction among blacks, researchers haven't been able to prove it. Dr. William Catalona, of Washington University, whose research status we've referred to earlier, now thinks race has little to do with the timing or frequency of Afro-American prostate cancers and that what appear to be racial differences stem instead from socioeconomic causes, delayed examinations, and lack of information.

Dr. Leslie R. Schover, Ph.D., staff psychologist at the Cleveland Clinic Foundation, a leading scholar and clinician in sex rehabilitation, told me that 41 to 63 percent (the range is from different studies) of men treated by radiation have some sexual dysfunction prior to treatment and that this may have led to overestimates of radiation as a cause of impotence. She said, "The prevalence may be closer to 25 percent of patients with new problems as opposed to the 50 percent often cited. . . . Men are more at risk to develop erection problems after radiotherapy if the quality of erections before treatment was borderline."

Recovery of potency after radical prostatectomy is better for younger patients when both neurovascular bundles can be spared and not quite so good if only one survives the surgery. (See Dr. Walsh's statistics on age and potency return in chapter 14, p. 102.)

Hormonal treatment affects the testicles' output of testosterone, the male sex hormone that acts in the brain to stimulate sexual desire and a man's ability to be aroused. Total androgen blockade also inhibits cancer cells from incorporating adrenal testosterone. Obviously, orchiectomy plus an antiandrogen does a similarly complete job. After or during hormonal treatment—orchiectomy or LHRH agonists (see chap. 15)—only about 20 percent of men remain sexually functional. The newer antiandrogens probably induce less of an effect but the jury is still out on those.

Dr. Schover caught my concentrated attention when she attacked the total problem of sexual capabilities and insisted that men (and women who have had various cancer treatments) need total rehabilitative counseling to improve their sex lives. She convinced me, too, when she told a San Francisco prostate cancer meeting that the statistics concerning potency after assorted treatments don't mean much. As you know, I am skeptical about a lot of the statistics concerning this disease.

The numbers tell us, for example, that after radiation probably half the patients eventually report a return of potency. The return may take six months to a year. The "nerve-sparing" surgeon, Dr. Patrick Walsh, asserts that, depending on their age, upwards of two-thirds of the men who have surgery in which the nerve–blood vessel packages on both sides of the prostate are saved can remain potent. Recovery of potency may take from six months to a year, sometimes two.

What Is Potency, Anyway?

But there's a lot more to it than these figures. What do they mean by potency? How many of these patients were potent before treatment? And just how potent were they and how potent are they now?

Generally, potency is defined as a man's ability to have an erection sufficient for vaginal penetration and to sustain it until climax and ejaculation, if he still has remaining after surgery the anatomical machinery for ejaculation. A man's degree of potency for the sake of the statistical reports is pretty much what he tells his doctor it is. His erection may be rigid, hard enough for thrusting. It may be semi-rigid, barely sufficient for penetration, or it may be semi-soft.

One doctor described the categories as "stickers and stuffers."

Stuffers don't thrust much and though they may consider themselves borderline potent they are limited in their action and in the positions they can
assume. The latter dysfunction may be frustrating to their partners. But,
after all, many of the men we're talking about forfeited their sexual acroba-
tic talents some years ago because of age, assorted impediments to blood
flow, such as smoking, diabetes, or other ailments. Besides, the women will
be glad their men are alive, still have fingers and mouths, and are concerned for their pleasure. (So I am authoritatively informed.)

One thing that screws up the statistics is that we tend to fib a lot. This
practice leads to less-than-accurate reports by doctors about their patients.
One doctor told me that he asked a patient how often he had sex. "Oh,
about once a week," the gray-head replied. The patient's wife, sitting on a
sofa behind him, looked the doctor in the eye and shook her head vigorously from side to side.

We know that men with less advanced stages of prostate cancer are
more likely to have a radical prostatectomy and those with more advanced
cancers, such as C's and worse, are more likely to undergo radiotherapy or
hormonal ablation. Also, patients selected for nerve-sparing surgical procedures are those considered better prospects, men with less probability of
tumor extended into the margins of the upcoming operation, younger, and
as a group in good health. Thus, comments Dr. Schover, it is not surprising
that a high percentage of such patients report good erections after their
treatment.

She also disagrees with the generally, and loosely, used figure of 50
percent for retention of erectile capacity following external beam radiotherapy. She calculates a higher figure, perhaps 75 percent, but—and this
is the critical point—she is including only men who had good erections
before treatment. Probably somewhere around 35 to 40 percent of those
headed for the LINAC are totally or partially impotent before they submit
to the beams.

In those whose function was borderline before radiotherapy and
among those who were smokers or had impaired penile circulation before
treatment the condition will be worse. Of men with rigid erections and approximately three incidents of activity per month prior to treatment, one
study showed, 73 percent managed good erections at eight- to twelve-
month follow-ups following radiation. Sometimes radiation may reduce
testosterone levels, but normal levels return in six to twelve months.

Hormonal therapy—orchiectomy, LHRH agonists, or combination
antiandrogens—costs most patients their potency and a loss of desire for
sex. Most have difficulty reaching orgasm even with prolonged sexual
stimulation, as Dr. Schover puts it. Younger patients, maybe 10 to 20 per-

cent, retain enough desire to initiate sex and manage adequate erections for the purpose. Treatment with LHRH agonists (Lupron, etc.) resulted in approximately the same loss of potency as other hormonal treatments. She urged further studies to find to what degree age or time in treatment affect sexual function.

More study is needed also on the effect of antiandrogens such as flutamide or nilutamide when used alone. These seem far less likely to reduce desire or capacity. No one clearly understands why androgen-blocking drugs might impair sexual function less than other types of hormonal therapy. In general, Dr. Schover found that hormonal therapy has a more "profound effect" on sexual desire than surgery or radiotherapy because of hormonal action on the brain, reducing desire and arousability. However, some men on antiandrogens were able to get erections through intense sexual fantasizing and those with especially strong motivation frequently were able to stay sexually active.

The sum of Dr. Schover's, and others', reports certainly is that the younger the patient and the more vigorous his sexual action prior to treatment the better the odds that he will emerge with his abilities, if not intact, at least serviceable. For those not prepared to wait out normal recovery time, if otherwise qualified for the therapy, radioactive seeds implantation may be an option.

Dr. Schover reported that many men think cancer is contagious and give up sexual activity out of fear of giving cancer to their partner. Prostate cancer cannot be given to someone else, certainly not women who have no prostate to begin with. Cancer cells in any event cannot be "transplanted" to another person through sexual contact. This is not AIDS. Some men even think of their cancer as punishment for past sexual activities.

The fear of losing sexual powers adds to the emotional impact of a prostate cancer diagnosis. A man may feel a loss of self-esteem and his positive feelings about his own body may decline. After treatment, if these fears are confirmed, a man may suffer severe depression and as a result lose his desire for sex altogether. She notes this is a particularly difficult confrontation for men who belong to ethnic groups that place high value on sexual performance as a mark of manhood.

The whole gamut of items that affect our sexual psyche becomes disordered with cancer treatments. Men may have to learn to deal with a dry orgasm following a radical prostatectomy. Several writers confirm that the sensation of intercourse and of orgasm is not adversely affected, but there will be no ejaculate. Following a transurethral resection, most men will have retrograde ejaculation and their perception will be one of a dry orgasm. Actually the ejaculate goes into the bladder which could care less.

The good news is that there are several possible therapies that can solve the erectile function problem. Another positive finding is that usually external genital sensations do not change and depending on your attitudes and remaining libido various indulgences up to the point of actual penile insertion might make up for some of your deprivation.

Dr. Schover urges studies concerning retention not only of "potency," but effective potency. She cites a study that questioned erectile quality after preservation of one neurovascular bundle. It reported that of twenty of twenty-nine men referred to as "potent" in follow-ups, only nine said their erection was of normal rigidity. Said Dr. Schover, in our interview:

> Some men are undoutedly satisfied with erections that are not fully rigid, but others may be frustrated by limitations on coital position, ease of thrusting, or the woman's pleasure when erections are barely functional. Should these men be offered intercavernous injections or vacuum erection devices during the first year after surgery when recovery of erections is often incomplete? Would such treatment have a positive or negative impact on ultimate recovery of erectile rigidity? Are we giving men inaccurate expectations about recovery of sexual function by defining a nonrigid erection as "potency"? What about other aspects of sexual function, i.e., desire for sex, penile sensation, ability to reach orgasm, quality of orgasm without semen? . . . these issues should be included in research protocols.[1]

What goes through the minds of men and their wives or partners following prostate cancer treatment? Most couples weather the changes in their sex life. Those in more recent or troubled relationships, however, may experience poor communication. Among couples who have been married for a long time divorce is rare. Dr. Schover is a strong advocate of counseling, for both partners. She says, "The challenge of the 1990s is the implementation of sexual rehabilitation programs that are practical, economic, and effective." And she's not speaking only of restoring firmer erections, or if the woman has been treated for cancer, overcoming *dyspareunia* (painful sexual intercourse). She defines rehabilitation as "remediation of the emotional impact of cancer diagnosis and treatment on body image, relationship satisfaction, and reproductive capacity."

She writes: "After cancer treatment, men may need longer foreplay and more direct penile stimulation to achieve the fullest possible erection. For some couples, intercourse may no longer be possible because erections are not rigid enough. If the couple has never engaged in manual or oral stimulation to the point of orgasm in the past, suggesting such alternatives to lovemaking is often futile."

Outside the major centers, specific sexual counseling is rarely available. Dr. Schover's writing is clear and nontechnical. She would not post it as a substitute for counseling, but I recommend it for men for whom counseling is not available or as a self-briefing prior to counseling. For physicians and counselors, she suggests a series of questions of the patient that can help reveal anxieties and focus rehabilitative strategies.

Restoring Your Erection, If You Want to

A man's erection is his own creation. In some societies it is a symbol of manhood, of virility. The phallic symbol appears in art and literature not only as a sexual icon but to evoke ideas of strength and honor. And, yes, this symbolism may not please the more aggressive feminists, although I've not heard of any action group objecting to the usage. A lot depends on built-in attitudes, I suppose. To some people, the Washington Monument is a phallic symbol. Yet the fact remains that many men see a loss of erections as a loss of manhood.

To understand some of the diagnostic procedures for determining potency and the use of various injections and prostheses for handling potency, let's examine the theories on the physiology of an erection.

Arterial blood flow is the prime mover. As an erection begins, nerve-transmitted messages relax the smooth muscles in the corpora cavernosa (those spongy tissue cylinders along each side of the penis).

These tissue spaces enlarge and the blood flow into them increases markedly. The small veins that normally drain these areas become squeezed between the expanding soft tissue and the muscular tissue at the base of the penis. This decreases the flow of blood away from the penis, it grows in diameter and length, and as blood pressure builds in the cavernosa it becomes rigid. When these small veins do not constrict and fail to stop the outflow of venous blood the problem is called venous leakage. The erection fails. There are constriction rings that will prevent this from happening. Some doctors may suggest a pony-tail holder or a rubber band at the base of the penis to serve as a temporary tourniquet to hold blood in the penis. Dr. Schover counters this advice with an emphatic no-no, noting that it can lead to edema (swelling) and the emergency room. Besides, such constrictors are usually useless. Devices for this purpose should be used under your doctor's supervision and should be easy to open. A proper ring usually comes with a vacuum erectile aid, if you buy one.

Drs. Walsh (see chapter 14, on surgery) and Pieter J. Donker, in their breakthrough studies back in 1982—the studies that lead to development of nerve-sparing surgery—found normal blood flow in a high percentage of impotent postoperative patients. They found through interviews that normal nighttime (while sleeping) penile tumescence did not occur in these men. With tremendous anatomical detail, they concluded that impotence after radical prostatectomies resulted from injury to the "pelvic nerve plexus" that directs the innervation of the corpora cavernosa.

They delineated two distinct pathways, neural (nerves) and psychic (the mind), that lead to increased arterial blood flow to the penis. One is a center that responds to mental stimulation. The other is a lumbar (in the lower back) sympathetic center that responds to direct penile stimuli. Also, branches of the pudendal nerve in the area just above the penis that do not travel through the "pelvic plexus" carry vital sensory perceptions from the skin of the penis.

That's enough of the mechanics. Just thinking through all this tangle of nerves, blood vessels, and the phenomenon of the unconscious mind's controlling one's erection may be sufficient to cause temporary impotence at some critical juncture in what is really a partnership process, with a real partner or a fantasized one.

Several manufacturers of devices to aid erections distribute pamphlets about their products with information concerning potency.[2] One says about 10 percent of the adult male population of the United States is impotent because of diabetes mellitus, vascular disease, prostate cancer treatments, various spinal injuries and other traumas, endocrine problems, or multiple sclerosis. Prostate treatments are responsible for 13 percent of that total, according to a variety of reports from assorted health agencies.

Most of us don't enjoy discussing this problem, even if it is our own. If we decide to attack it with the idea of curing it or circumventing it, we'll have various tests, including a psychological screening because most of us, again, don't want to acknowledge the stress, frustration, possible embarrassment, or even fear that, depending on our ages and relationships, impotence engenders.

Healthy men will have three to five erections while sleeping at night. These occur during what is known as REM (rapid eye movement) cycles of sleep. There are at least two systems for monitoring these. One is a ring type device that goes around the penis before you go to bed. It has small filaments in it that, should nighttime erections occur, will break. A more sophisticated method attaches to a monitor connected to rings around the penis. It will measure all penis activity, including frequency of erections, erectile quality, and duration. Arterial blood flow can be measured, as can nerve conductivity. This is a laboratory drill, not generally available.

Unfortunately, our prostate brethren already know their problem although they might want to know more specifics about it. If blood flow is OK, an injection of papaverine, among other drugs, in the penis will produce an erection. Indeed, such injections are one solution to regaining an erection on demand.

Other tests may be made by ultrasound to "picture" blood vessel conditions below the skin. An injection is used to assess the size of penile arteries. Something called "dynamic infusion cavernosometry" gauges fluid pressure changes and the speed of blood flow with an erection in the penis, again produced by injections of medication. This test measures both arterial and venous flow. I add that all this involves assorted clinicians observing and handling what you've undoubtedly considered in the past an intimate part of your body, not to be casually submitted to such persistent investigations. Obviously, some men are able to place the goal they hope to achieve above the intrusions.

Erections can be generated with injections, vacuum devices that in effect pull blood into the penis, and with a variety of surgically implanted devices. Injections usually are of papaverine, phentalomine, or prostaglandin E1. Your urologist will teach you how to inject the drug into your penis. An extremely fine needle is employed. The medication is sold in 10 cc lots. Costs vary according to the type and concentration of the medicine but say, roughly, $10 or up a shot. It must be kept under refrigeration. The drugs must be obtained by prescription and are only carried by special pharmacies. A dose consists usually of one-half a cc and may be administered as often as three times a week. Some programs limit injections to two a week. Some men with more vascular obstruction may need larger doses.

The only requirement is that you can learn to give yourself the injection and have the manual dexterity to do it. Dr. Schover suggests that "a committed spouse can learn to give the injection." The injection is given, or taken, some fifteen to thirty minutes before intercourse and the resultant erection may last from one to three hours.

Episodes of "priapism," meaning a painful erection that will not go away for extended periods, do not happen often with the doses your doctor will recommend, after some tests. But the condition is an emergency and requires fast medical attention, as it can cause severe damage to blood vessels. The affliction gets its name from Priapus, a Greek god associated with phallic worship. He was reputed to be an ugly devil, though extravagantly endowed, the son of Dionysius and Aphrodite, and was celebrated by various cults, frequently with orgies. Anyway, the dosage has to be accurate. Don't experiment yourself.

Patients start with very small doses after learning how to draw the drug into the needle. The dosage may be gradually increased. Prolonged use of papaverine or phentalomine can cause penile fibrosis which would be similar to scar tissue or a hardening of connective tissues. In programs at

Cleveland Clinic, Dr. Schover noted a smaller but still significant rate of fibrosis with prostaglandin E1. The men sometimes suffered curvature of the penis. Consequently, men on these intercavernous injections should have regular examinations. The curvatures may be the result, or even an exacerbation, of Peyronie's disease, cause unknown, which is a thickening of the fibrous tissues within the penis forcing it to bend at an angle during erection. Usually it affects only one side and can make intercourse painful or impossible. Also with prostaglandin E1 about a third to a half of the men injected will feel burning for a few minutes after the injection and may not like the effect.

Dr. Nash considers the injection treatments satisfactory, especially for use shortly after surgery. "Say I have a patient who is forty-nine. We're confident that in a year he'll be as potent as he was before, but if we're talking about three months after surgery, why wait? We'll put him on injections until he can function without them." Other urologists share his sentiment and prescribe either vacuum devices or injections during the first year after surgery. Apparently this does not interfere with eventual recovery of unaided erectile ability.

Some of Dr. Nash's patients have used the injections for as long as seven years, one for eight. One of the vacuum device firms says thirty thousand men are using one or the other of the injection medications, which are said to be not very painful. Yet Dr. Nash finds some patients get impatient and annoyed with the injections and request penile implants.

Then there are medicines known as "vasodilators." They can dilate arteries and increase blood flow. One is nitroglycerine ointment. Nitro frequently is used in treating high blood pressure and heart problems. Applied to the penis it may improve erection, but it frequently causes headaches and is easily absorbed by the vagina, so you must wear a condom to avoid giving your partner a headache, which would be a poor present in exchange for what she is doing for you. Given possible side effects and a lack of true scientific study of this procedure, the real effectiveness may be marginal and many men don't get good erections from it, anyway.

Taken by tablet, probably three a day, Yohimbine seems to have helped 20 to 25 percent of its users restore reasonably serviceable erections. Some 60 percent report partial but noticeable improvement after about eight weeks of treatment, which, if it has worked at all, must be continued or impotence may return. It is made from the bark of the Yohimbe tree, which grows in India and Africa and has reputed aphrodisiac properties. It is supposed to have a salutary effect on nerves that might inhibit an erection. It might also increase libido in some. It might cause some mild dizziness or headaches, irritability, increased heart rate, or skin flushing, but apparently these effects are minimized when it is taken with meals. It should not be used by men with tendencies toward gastric or duodenal ulcers nor in company with antidepressant drugs of any kind. It has been found not to be effective for impotence following a radical prostatectomy. Furthermore, its help if any is probably psychological, like a placebo.

A Mr. Geddings Osbon Sr. started a foundation devoted to impotency study with money earned from a device called ErecAid. It is one of a number of external vacuum therapies. The penis is placed in a plastic tube connected to a small hand operated pump that withdraws air from the tube. The vacuum created draws blood into the penis. ErecAid has counselors (very low-pressure sales people) who teach men to use the device and to increase their erections gradually, not try to pump up to some macho size immediately. There is a tension ring of plastic or rubber that, once an erection is achieved, slides off the cylinder and around the base of the penis to prevent venous leakage and thus maintain the erection which lasts about thirty minutes. The band should not be worn for more than thirty minutes.

More than fifty thousand men use or have used external vacuum devices either for continued impotence therapy or as a temporary aid before surgical corrective procedures. Men whose penile implants have been removed may use a vacuum device. The devices earn a good rate of approval and even help restore normal erections sometimes. The tension ring must be exactly the right size or either the erection won't be maintained or ejaculation may be painful, if ejaculatory powers remain effective. Users report general satisfaction in spite of the fact that foreplay must be interrupted for the application. The counselors advise that one train his partner to assist in the process. Your doctor will set up an appointment for you with a representative of a vacuum device company. You must have a prescription to buy one. The cost is about $400.

Dr. Schover's research reports that the vacuum-induced erection may be larger in circumference than the natural one and, "unfortunately," she writes, "is often not firm right next to the constriction band, so that the penis pivots, which can interfere with thrusting during intercourse." The ErecAid company reported their drop-out rate is only about 20 percent, which attests either to the value of the procedure or to some men's lack of concern over getting their $400 back. Clinicians think the drop-out rate for vacuum pumps may be as high as 50 percent the first year.

There are several different models of penile prostheses available. All must be surgically inserted into the erectile chambers of the penis. These devices produce a high rate of success, about 90 percent. Intercourse can be started four to six weeks after the surgery.

The simplest device is a semi-rigid or malleable rod. The implantation is relatively simple, produces few complications, and is the least expensive of the inserts. The penis is erect all the time, however, and so this implant, which we might call the "ready teddy," may sometimes be difficult to conceal. Or, it might get you a lot of offers, depending on the circles you travel in. It is made to be bent out of the way, somewhat.

Probably the best system, in that it more closely simulates normal erectile activity, is the fully inflatable insert. There are two types of these. One type is made up of two cylinders surgically implanted in the penis and connected to a pumping mechanism, with a fluid reservoir, located in the abdomen or the scrotum. The devices are activated by gently squeezing or pressing the inflation pump. This pumps fluid to the balloon cylinders and brings the penis to attention. A release valve returns the penis to rest. The failure rate with the newest of such devices is low, about 3 percent within the first three years of use. On the downside, but rarely, scar tissue can form around the reservoir or the pump, the cylinders can leak or break, and the connecting tubing can become obstructed. However, in most of the insertions the newer designs of implants work flawlessly for years.

Another type is also a two-piece implant, a simpler installation since there is no separate fluid reservoir. This avoids the need to install a reservoir elsewhere. It consists of two inflatable rods, one on either side of the penis. Each rod has its own pump and its own inflate-deflate mechanism built in. It is activated by squeezing the pump at the tip of the penis.

Most implantations usually require only a small incision. Some surgeons do them on an outpatient basis. Most install them under a general or spinal anaesthetic with a one- to two-day hospital stay.

These various implants differ in cost. For the most complex, the price is about $3,500 depending on your hospital's mark-up. For the package—device, surgery, anaesthesia, hospital—the whole shooting match will run from $7,500 to $10,000, often as high as $15,000. Some hospitals won't allow implants: they feel the equipment vendors' prices are too high and it costs the hospital to yield a reasonable rate to the patient. Recently, Medicare payments have failed to meet the full cost of the device, the hospital, and the surgery.

Moreover, each of the implant devices produces slightly different results in terms of the girth or length of the erection. And each has its own medical requirements, related to whether you were treated by radiation or a radical prostatectomy. Another point to bring up with your urologist.

Your doctor may be able to suggest some prostate brothers willing to talk to you about their implants and pass along more personal knowledge.

Or you might agree with a couple inquiring about an implant who was told the cost would be about $10,000. They asked for a day or two to think it over, called the doctor and declined. "We think we'd rather redo the kitchen," the wife said.

The point is that if continued sexual activity is important to you and your partner there are ways you can continue it almost unabated, with most of the sensations intact. If you can handle all this yourself, with your doctor, you are a particularly self-contained and confident person. Good counseling, if not for you, for your wife and you together, is an option that could prove rewarding. Most of us handle sex better than we handle conversation about sex.

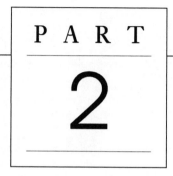

PART

2

Direct from the Doc

The Important Questions for You to Ask Your Doctor

YOU WILL FIND A NUMBER of easy to read and understand pamphlets useful in starting your education in prostate cancer. Your doctor will probably give you some from the American Cancer Society. There's a national organization of support groups named Us Too, very young but growing swiftly. Unfortunately, it expects an increasing number of prospects for membership.

Several physicians have written their own informative bulletins for patients. In their simplistic and introductory way, these pamphlets weren't enough. I want detail. I want the whats and the whys answered in depth.

Many men hesitate to go to a doctor for prostate exams because they think treatment will affect their sexual capacities and that's frequently not true. When is it not true? Which treatments might offer the better chances of preserving potency and what might restore it, if it is lost? If I am to be in a battle, I want to know the enemy. Familiarity and knowledge, to me, make enduring the disease easier; doubts and misapprehensions might be dispelled if I learn what "it is like" to go through the experience.

Several medical points of contention flourish in this field, which has received more attention in the past ten years than in all previous clinical history. The application of new diagnostic technologies is triggering the discovery explosion statisticians anticipated. New cases in 1993, about 165,000, were up 22 percent over 1992. Upwards of 200,000 are expected in 1994. The doctors are thinking more and more about the quality of life a patient might anticipate, depending on the stage of his cancer, following one treatment as compared to another, and are judging their therapies accordingly, as well as considering what will keep you alive the longest.

With the quantity and pace of research increasing, are we better qualified to make a choice between radiation and surgical therapies, for example?

Which of the new treatment methods best fits our personal mindset as well as our personal cancer?

Because there are no quick cures, even to the benign problems the prostate invokes, and because there are so many variations on the prostate cancer theme, the doctor stands as the all-knowing overseer of that marvelous machinery of reproduction and waste disposal combined in your lower abdomen. He will be the guru in your life who comprehends this concatenation of conduits with their little input stations of lubricants and nutrients along their production line. He feels them from the outside, probes them from the inside and peers at them even through the wall of skin and muscle around them with assorted rays and scans and dyes and even sound. You will think of him when thou risest up (probably to pee) and when thou liest down (several times in the night) and when he toucheth you where the sun don't shine.

Moreover, he's getting better at his tasks. Advances in screening and posttreatment diagnosis through blood tests, in the technology and techniques of radiotherapy, in advances in surgical procedures and in hormonal treatments, even in applications of subzero temperatures, improve his chances of not only keeping you alive and functioning but of curing you altogether.

Hard-Nosed Counsel on Selecting Your Physician, and Questions You Might Ask

Even in my brief acquaintance with prostate cancer I've talked to patients whose postoperative troubles and misdiagnosed problems convince me, not to blame the profession across the board, but to be aware that physicians like the rest of us have their biases, their beliefs in their own omniscience, and their pet absolutes which are not always applicable to every patient.

I am impressed by Dr. Nash's directness and blunt authority in explaining to patients their precise medical condition. He has reviewed this manuscript for medical accuracy and guided me through the twists and tangents of articles in medical journals. He's seen enough, read enough, conferred enough to have developed firm convictions about what patients should know so they can share in the major decisions involved in their own treatment.

So the counsel that follows for the next several pages is direct from the doctor, untouched by journalistic hands. First is his general advice; then, a series of questions that suggest what you might ask your physician for fuller understanding of our problem. These are important first steps you should take to discover disease, if any, early enough to beat it, and strategies you should consider seriously if you need treatment.

Pay Heed

Memo from Seymour C. Nash, M.D., Fellow, American College of Surgeons; Diplomate, American Board of Urology:

1. Beginning in your fortieth year, have a PSA (prostatic specific antigen blood serum test) annually. If your grandfather, father, brother, or uncle had a cancer of the prostate, have the test twice a year. Any change in the series over the extent of the tests raises strong suspicion of prostate cancer.

2. Have a yearly or semi-yearly digital (finger) rectal exam by an expert, someone who does the test frequently and knows what he's feeling. This means a urologist, not a general practitioner or an internist or a cardiologist. Go for experience. Until the PSA test came along, I received almost no referrals from general practitioners who "felt something in the prostate." Most don't know if they are feeling anything or not.

3. If an elevated PSA or a suspicious DRE (digital rectal exam) means you require a transrectal ultrasound procedure, research the doctor who will perform the U/S (ultrasound) test. How often does he do them? How long has he been doing them? What machine does he use? Is he using the latest equipment? Does he do the tests himself or have a technician do them for him? Does he do his own biopsies (take tissue samples for lab examinations)? If the early tests are negative and he is still suspicious, does he do random biopsies in addition to aiming his biopsy needle at a target revealed by ultrasound (U/S)?

4. If your PSA is elevated or if something is seen on the U/S screen, your prostate should be biopsied and there should be some random biopsies taken away from the precise site of suspicious images on the U/S. If your PSA is elevated, you should have random biopsies even if the U/S picture shows nothing. Remember this: 17 to 30 percent of cancers of the prostate will not elevate your PSA; up to 30 percent of cancers cannot be felt in a DRE. Indeed, cancer may be multifocal, that is in several locations, and not be detected by U/S. Both sides of your prostate should be biopsied, always, even if one side or the other shows nothing in the ultrasound scan.

5. If your biopsies are found to contain cancer, you should be clinically *staged* (categorized) with bone and CT scans, perhaps an endorectal MRI (magnetic resonance imaging with a probe up the rectum). If these scans are negative, the lymph nodes that drain your prostate may have to be evaluated to see if cancer has spread to them. This can be done either at the time of an operation for removal of your prostate or prior to radiation ther-

apy (either external or with implanted "seeds") or cryosurgery. This exam may be done *laparoscopically*, a relatively newer and easier-on-the-patient surgical procedure than was used in the past. If your Gleason grade is high, in the 7–10 range, or your PSA is above 20, you are more likely to have a positive finding of cancer in your lymph nodes and/or bones.

Although many radiologists treat patients without knowing the status of the lymph nodes, you should insist on this exam or you will not know the true extent of your disease, or insist on an explanation of why you should not have it. This is new stuff: probably your friends who may have been treated even as recently as one or two years ago did not have node exams before radiation. If tumor is in your lymph nodes, your treatment will be modified.

6. If there is tumor in your lymph nodes, you will require hormonal blockade, that is, complete suppression of your body's male hormones. This requires an *orchiectomy* (removal of the testicles), or monthly treatment with drugs such as Lupron (that accomplish the same thing, but much more expensively), plus an antiandrogen, e.g., flutamide. Lupron checks the body's production of testicular testosterone; flutamide the uptake of other testosterone, including adrenal.

7. If your biopsy is negative you could still have cancer and should be followed with periodic DRE's and PSA tests. You may also need additional biopsies.

8. If your PSA continues to climb in the absence of rectal findings, your tumor could be hiding from the finger or the rise could be caused by a low grade inflammation and you should be on antibiotics for a time to see if the PSA decreases. If after multiple biopsies no cancer is found and the PSA remains high you may need a *transurethral resection* (TURP) in which tissue is removed from the prostate through the penis for diagnosis.

9. Recently, the matter of *prostatic specific antigen density* has arisen as a diagnostic tool and is useful in interpreting PSA readings. The density is obtained by dividing the PSA level by the weight of the prostate, in grams (determined ultrasonically). Ask about it.

10. Your biopsy may not find cancer but could show a pre-malignant lesion called PIN that is associated with cancer. The high grade type of PIN indicates a cancer elsewhere in the gland, meaning more biopsies will be required, or augurs a future cancer. Its diagnostic use is relatively new.

Your urologist will discuss all this with you. He should discuss some of the newer techniques and machines, such as color doppler ultrasound that can indicate cancer in areas not usually seen because they are concealed by other internal elements of your body. These new machines may be a major wave of the future in prostate cancer diagnosis.

If you have a localized cancer, which means confined to the prostate, you should have a complete health evaluation with input from your cardiologist: echo tests, cardiogram, stress thalium tests, a total workup. If you are otherwise in good health and have a life expectancy longer than ten years you may have to make a decision concerning whether you want to be treated surgically, by radiation, or with cryosurgery. Your urologist will recommend a procedure, but he will want you to decide. The "watching and waiting" course is not for patients with early disease who have a ten-year life expectancy and who want to be cured. To "watch and wait" may insure your incurability. This book explores the factors that will help you make this decision.[1]

Interviewing Your Doctor

Here are some questions I suggest you ask a urologist in determining whether you will put your life in his hands.

1. Does he treat all prostate cancer patients with radiotherapy and refer them to a radiotherapist?

2. If surgery is the choice, does your urologist operate on all patients himself? If so, how many procedures does he do each year? Are his treatments tailored to each patient? Know his thinking before you commit to him. If you may have surgery, ask him how frequently he operates and what complications he has experienced. Ask how much blood he uses and how long it takes him to do the job.

3. Speak to his other patients. Confer with nurses or anesthesiologists. Use any friends or connections you have with your hospital to learn what other health professionals think of your surgeon. Get as many opinions as you can and try to make sure they are not tainted. It is important to know if your urologist does surgery, if he does it himself, or if he sends most patients out for radiation.

4. If using radiation, does he advise doing it by external beam or by implanted seeds or by a combination of the two? Ask questions about possible complications. Ask about the experience of the "providers," and their track records. Don't be timid. All radiotherapists and urologists are not equal: training, experience, and mindsets vary. These factors are a big part of the reason for successes and failures in treatment. Are implanted seeds available in your hospital? (You will better understand the answer after you read chapter 12, part 1.)

5. Ask the physicians advising you to tell you about meetings and conferences they have attended on cancer of the prostate and try to find how open-minded they are. Changes occur swiftly in this field and your advisors should be current on new therapies and modifications of standard ones.

6. Find out if your treatment is part of a study and make sure you are not a unit. Studies are going on at many universities and centers and unwillingly and unknowingly you may find your treatment altered to fit the study parameters.[2]

7. Do some research on your advisor. Don't go to a general medical oncologist except for an opinion on your potential surgeon or radiotherapist. The generalist may be well behind the times as far as prostate cancer is concerned. If you go to an oncologist, go to a specialist in prostate cancer. Remember, your internist or cardiologist may refer you, with all good intentions, to a friend and really not know if he is the best qualified.

8. Just because a person is a professor or head of a department does not mean he has the best qualifications to do a hands-on radical operation. I personally know of a consumer who decided to go to a particular hospital because he had strong ties to it and his cardiologist was there. The urology professor at this hospital had just completed an observational course on the type of surgery he intended to do on the patient but was not experienced at it. He took over three times the usual time and eight times the usual amount of blood in the procedure. Research your providers as much as you can.

9. What is the doctor's follow-up plan after your initial treatment? After radiation therapy or surgery you should be followed primarily by your urologist, who will periodically take PSA's, do rectal exams, and order other evaluative tests as needed. By way of explanation, you can have residual carcinoma of the prostate and still have a negative rectal exam. For years patients were followed by radiotherapists and oncological urologists with rectal exams only. That alone may be a useless procedure. With the advent of PSA and transrectal ultrasound, evaluations can be more accurate. Re-biopsy may be necessary after a year or two if your PSA does not follow the proper postradiation treatment trend or if your rectal exam is suspicious.

10. Ask about test procedures: Does he do them himself? What equipment does he use? What is his experience with it?

11. Is he keeping up to date? What conferences has he attended lately? Ask about trends in diagnosis and treatment.

If your PSA does not fall to negligible levels after surgery, or if it rises, you may need radiation therapy, also. If there are signs of local spread, that is, cancer remaining in the margins around where your prostate used to be, you will need postoperative radiation therapy. So your doctor should have a plan that will assure you of continued care and assessment of your condition.—SCN

The Time Bomb Itself

Where and What Is the Prostate and What Does It Do?

PROSTATE CANCER IS A SERIOUS DISEASE and contending with it will occupy a sizeable chunk of your lives.

We tend to think of the prostate as the ultimate male chauvinist topic, for men only. It is strictly a male organ and does not directly contact the other gender, as do other male organs we might mention. However, the prostate does function necessarily in the reproductive process in that it produces the fluid that nourishes and transports sperm to its destination. Intercourse is possible without your prostate: you just can't make babies.

Neither is the prostate patient alone with his sexual and other problems, as this disease does not enhance the lives of those around him, especially in cases of advanced disease. Cornelius Ryan, the author of *The Longest Day* and *Bridge Too Far* wrote in detail of his long and losing struggle with prostate cancer. His desperate searching ranged him across this country, Europe, and Asia seeking cures. His eventual decline into total dependency on his family exhausted him and them. When he finally died, it was a blessed relief to them despite their grief.

I do not give medical advice. That's a doctor's job. But when friends call, I do steer them, with Dr. Nash's help, to where sound advice may be obtained.

One such call came from a woman friend, long divorced and now living in California. Now in her early sixties, she found herself deeply in love with a man of approximately her own age. They had decided to marry. The discovery shortly afterwards that he had cancer of the prostate shocked them and forced a reappraisal of their plans. She explained that they were sexually active and that sex was an important part of their relationship. If treatment were to render him impotent, she agonized, she did not want a sexless marriage.

Furthermore, she did not want the responsibility after years of being single and at her age of caring for an invalid. I could not advise her specifically and I suspected that sex, love, and the man were inseparable in her mind, an understandable situation. We suggested several excellent doctors and clinics in her part of the country. I later learned he had a PSA of 40 and underwent radiation treatment. A year later they were still together and seemed quite happy, and he is doing well. So far this story is going nicely but the anxiety and tension that developed on the way to a contented conclusion does demonstrate that men usually are not alone with this problem.

Wives and families become deeply distressed when a disease appears with "cancer" in its name. Loss or interruption of sexual activity may not be as important to some as to others but in most families wives and children do not want their husbands and fathers to suffer, perhaps die. They want to do something helpful and caring but they don't know what that might be. And, often as not, old dad appears as healthy and lively as ever. He even feels good and frequently reacts with annoyance to an excess of solicitude.

Of course, your wife will be concerned. She will ask if you should have a special diet, if you are taking your medicine (although there might be none to take at this point). When is your next test? What does it mean? That sudden passing pain in your hip—is it the cancer? (Unless the cancer is advanced, it's probably a little arthritis, aggravated by a bad golf swing.)

It is wise to share with family all the knowledge available about the illness, the good and the bad: not to frighten them but to gain mutual understanding. This will not be easy if the disease progresses despite treatment. Counselors are available to help these relationships.

Supportive Organizations—or the Lack Thereof

The popular press addresses the prostate only when a celebrity discloses his problem or when some related medical advance arises. Until we are involved the information doesn't sink in. Neither does it arise in general conversation and those who aren't aware of prostate dangers think they don't want to hear about them. (Though they should.) The prostate is not among those organs given to romantic and/or threatening public awareness campaigns. I have never been invited to a rubber chicken dinner to be importuned for funds to fight prostate cancer. I found no nationwide fund-raising foundation exclusively devoted to prostate research until recently, when the director of the Mathews Foundation for Prostate Research, Ms. Mary Lou Wright, wrote an article that appeared in several newspapers. Founded in 1988, the Mathews Foundation is still modestly endowed compared to more venerable single purpose foundations. Mostly it underwrites or shares research costs in California institutions.[1]

The American Cancer Society includes prostatic cancer in its portfolio. The National Institutes of Health does also through its National Cancer Institute. Several specific research organizations within these groups concentrate on prostate cancer, but not until early 1991, when the American Foundation for Urologic Disease (AFUD) was formed, was there a general organization—not doctors only—formed targeted to urological diseases, including prostate problems.[2]

The Prostate Itself

Shortly after my own prostate cancer was diagnosed I played poker in my old hometown, Gainesville, Ga., with five other men about my own age (sixty-nine) whom I have known for more than forty years. To my surprise, I discovered three of them had had prostate cancer therapies within the past year: two had surgery and one radiation. They felt fine. I didn't ask about their sex lives; I'm not that brash a reporter.

Some time later at a luncheon in Miami attended by about three hundred people, mostly men, I spoke with a friend in his mid-eighties whom I hadn't seen for a while and when he asked how I'd been I told him. "Join the club," he said. "I had prostate cancer surgery fifteen years ago and I could point to twenty or more men in this room with prostate cancer wounds of one kind or another." So, when you become a novitiate in the fraternity of troubled prostates you find a lot of company. Frankly, I found it reassuring. After all, I saw a lot of survivors in that room. That crowd of graduates also was more convincing than bare statistics concerning the incidence of a group of diseases which, when you study them, still present an assortment of mysteries and debates to the medicine men. On the other hand, I didn't know how many of their contemporaries had died along the way, either.

These ruminations encouraged me to get down to business: just what is the prostate and what does it do?

Most men know that only males have prostates and that the prostate has something to do with their sex life, though exactly what they're not sure. Street jokes suggest that as men age, their prostate changes, usually enlarging, which is true, but the street assumption that prostate trouble means the end of one's sex life isn't necessarily true. Nonmalignant prostate problems rarely threaten potency and at least one such problem actually may be eased by increased sexual activity. The new nerve-sparing surgical techniques, especially with younger men, can leave unimpaired the nerves governing what doctors call "the erectile function."

The prostate is part of the genito-urinary complex of tubes, valves, and assorted fluid-secreting and -storage mechanisms involved in urination and reproduction.

The normal prostate is about the size of a chestnut, as doctors like to describe it, shaped somewhat like a pyramid, about an inch and a half to two inches at its widest. Normally, it weighs about 15 to 20 grams, although one doctor wrote that he once removed a prostate that weighed 275 grams. It resides next to the rectum, up about one or two inches from the anus, directly below the bladder. It sits directly above the very rear of the penis root over the first part of that spongy tissue called the corpora cavernosa. This mass of tissue extends over the scrotum and along the penis. It is what becomes engorged with blood to produce an erection.

The urethra, through which urine passes to be voided from the body, begins at the lower end of the bladder and runs through, or is surrounded by, the prostate, into the penis. The urethra is a tough little muscular tube which fortunately for us men is able to regenerate itself when it must be "cored out" to relieve the pressure on it from prostatic enlargement, which interferes mightily with urine flow.

The prostate resides just under the bladder and "in front" of the rectum. It surrounds the urethra as that tube passes into the penis. Not all of it can be felt by the physician in his digital rectal examination. This is one reason the DRE misses some tumors.

The prostate consists of five lobes, part glandular and part fibromuscular tissue, containing a bunch of little tubes, connected to fifteen or twenty small ducts lined with mucous membrane and surrounded by muscle, all contained in what is called the capsule. The prostate doesn't grow to "normal" size until puberty when male hormones awaken it. It starts growing again when a man reaches about fifty, though the medical literature isn't clear on why that happens. It may be part of a glandular syndrome roughly comparable to menopause in a woman. Possibly it reacts to changes in the male hormone testosterone.[3]

What does the prostate do and why do you need one? Its one definitive function, upon which all doctors agree, is to produce a fluid that transports and feeds sperm cells through their various developmental routes in the system and then carries the sperm through ejaculation. About 95 percent of the fluid in ejaculation is prostatic secretion (4 percent is fluid from the seminal vesicles and 1 percent is sperm and other fluids).

You can see it takes a lot of plumbing plus coordinated fluids to carry that sperm to where it can do its job. The prostate also produces some enzymes, maybe some hormones. Just what their functions may be isn't scientifically established.

Since a male whose prostate has been removed has almost never been known to impregnate a woman (though he may function in every other way), doctors believe the prostatic fluid is essential to the sperm's mission.

21

The Track of the Sperm
A Thirteen-Week Journey

SINCE WE ARE TRYING to understand the prostatic function and know more about systems related to it, the body's manufacture of sperm and how these potent little creatures get to their eventual destination applies. Combining various articles and descriptions of the process and clearing the medical technicalities out of the way, their travel goes like this:

Produced in the testicles, sperm matures in about ten weeks. Then it leaves the testicles and enters the epididymides, tube-like structures behind each testicle, and rests another three weeks. Then it goes to a sort of loop behind the bladder (vasa deferentia) and is stored in places called the ampullae which are next to sac-like glands called the seminal vesicles. These lie along the prostate and secrete a fluid (lactose or fructose) that nourishes the sperm while it waits for you to do with it what you are supposed to do. In your reading you may see sketches or diagrams of the prostate with what appear to be little wings along each side. These are the seminal vesicles and are quite susceptible to cancer cell invasion. Surgical removal of the prostate removes the seminal vesicles, too. Ejaculatory ducts go from the seminal vesicles through the prostate, taking on fluid from the prostate and also from Cowper's glands, two pea-sized glands on either side of the urethra. This mix of nutrients and fluids runs through the urethra and is ejaculated through the penis.

I mean, you may think you are just fooling around, fella, but you are in fact cranking up a complicated process. And, did you realize that the last time you released a crowd of them to do their will, they were already thirteen weeks old?

22

What Causes This Cancer?

Is It Something We Eat? Or Where We Work?

WHAT EVERY MAN ASKS: maybe something in the air or something I ate or didn't eat woke up this cancer. Answering the question, how and where did I get this frightening and troublesome invader? is easy for your reporter. The answer is, nobody knows.

For all the major impact of prostate cancer on millions of men in the world, you'd think the discovery and diagnosis of the disease, especially its causes, would have been well defined by now. Not so. New findings and applications crop up regularly. For example, more information appears periodically concerning the impact of diet and environment, especially in the workplace, on prostate cancer.

The heaviest suspicion currently falls on the fatty acids in red meats and certain oils such as soybean oil, not perhaps as the trigger for prostate cancer startup (tumorigenesis) but as a prime villain in stimulating a latent prostate cancer to grow to an advanced cancer. The details are in this chapter, but meanwhile, if you've been found to have a small cancer or are concerned about reawakening your already treated cancer you should consider ridding your diet of beef, lamb, pork, and chicken with skin. From my reading, were I in the "watch and wait" category, I'd watch and wait as a vegetarian except for fish and poultry, which I would eat skinless.

Prostate cancer is not a "you have it or you don't have it" problem. It is not liable to instant definition. This is not a broken leg or a clogged artery. It comes in a number of stages. It has a strong relationship to male hormones, responding to the body's production of testosterone so directly that a major area of treatment of advanced disease involves shutting down the body's testosterone utilization. Red meat, animal fats, and certain oils are thought to increase testosterone levels in the body. This is thought to be a major reason why there is more prostate cancer in countries where diets include a lot of meat and/or animal fats.

If you are a North American or European white, age forty or older, you are in high risk territory. If you are black in these geographies, your chance of having the disease is almost twice that of whites. In the rest of the world, rates of prostate cancer differ widely, with Oriental and eastern European countries having the lowest.

The age-specific prevalence of histologic evidence (meaning some cancer cells) is similar in Japanese and U.S. men but the clinical (meaning requiring treatment) incidence is significantly higher in the U.S.

Ruben F. Gittes, M.D., in the *New England Journal of Medicine* reported that the incidence of clinically diagnosed prostatic cancer ranged from 0.8 cases per 100,000 population in Shanghai, China, to 100.1 per 100,000 among blacks in Alameda County, California.[1] Geography aside, it is much more common among whites than Asians. Says Dr. Gittes,

> Several studies have indicated that the incidence of latent carcinoma at autopsy is similar in different ethnic groups. Since this would seem to eliminate a genetic basis for the appearance of latent prostatic carcinoma, what accounts for the disparate growth of these tiny tumors to clinically important size in different countries and races? An attractive but conjectural hypothesis is that it is the serum testosterone level, and since a vegetarian diet may [result in] lower serum testosterone levels, the combination of race and diet can predict some if not all of the epidemiological [geographic occurrence] spectrum of prostate cancer.

He urged further studies to test this theory. More recent studies tend to blame animal fat, as we shall see, rather than testosterone but the two are linked to some degree.

There is one area of certainty. It can be familial. The Brady Urological Institute at Johns Hopkins circulated a request to doctors for information on patients who may have inherited an abnormal gene from either parent. It urged physicians when taking family histories to include all men on both sides of the family—fathers, brothers, uncles, and grandfathers. It said if you have any relative who developed prostate cancer before age fifty-five, or two or more relatives with prostate cancer, you may be susceptible to the inherited form of the disease. Other doctors maintain that if you have a father and an uncle, or any two first-degree relatives, who had prostate cancer, your chances of developing it increase eightfold.

If you have only one relative with the disease, especially if he was over seventy at discovery, it is unlikely you have a high risk of inheriting the disease. Any man, checking his mother's as well as his father's relatives, should begin exams at age forty and advise his brothers and/or sons to do the same. Johns Hopkins hopes to identify the gene that carries the disease.

*   *   *

I've eaten all my life about what most everybody else in America eats. As a child, I ate what my mother put in front of me except for sneaked Milky Ways and too much bubble gum. In college with little time for breakfast I usually started the day with a large chocolate milkshake and a Moon Pie.[2] Otherwise, the usual; perhaps too many late-night hamburgers. In the Navy, I certainly consumed the standard fare also, including on a few occasions of temporary deprivation, too much Spam and powdered eggs. As an adult, I have thrived (except for THIS) on a non-exotic U.S. of A. diet: meat, potatoes, salad, iced tea, several cups of coffee (for the past ten years or so, de-caf only), and various desserts, not too many of those. In my high-pressure working days, my late afternoon pick-me-up was a Mr. Goodbar. Even into advanced adulthood, I favor a glass of milk (skimmed, these days) and a couple of chocolate cookies before bedtime. To my regret, newer research reports include fats in milk, including butter, as a possible provocateur in prostate country.

I've always liked vegetables, especially fresh ones prepared in the vaunted Southern style: buttered squash, fried okra, lima beans, green peas, black-eyes peas with butter and chopped onions, not quite ripe tomatoes. I've always disliked mayonnaise and learned early on how difficult it is in an eatery to order and receive a BLT with mustard instead of mayonnaise. I'm the only person I know who regularly sends BLT's back to be re-slathered.

My meat consumption consists mostly of lean beef, lamb chops, and sometimes veal; infrequently, bacon at breakfast. Anne and I rarely have pork, not for religious reasons but because we don't like it very much. Chicken we eat a lot of, especially fried. Our home town of Gainesville, Ga., ranks as one of the major poultry producing centers of the entire world and anyone there who professed not to like chicken might as well publicly confess to membership in a Satanic cult. And to peel the crunchy skin off fried chicken before eating it would mark one as a definitely peculiar person, maybe even a Yankee! (Nevertheless, the skin should come off.)

I've always been a light drinker. I found early that a slight excess of alcohol makes me nauseous. One cold martini at eventide, however, is a welcome treat.

So what did me in? Too many french fries? Chicken fat? OD-ing on bittersweet dark chocolate? Lots of cocoa-fat in chocolate. Not enough broccoli?

Perhaps something in the environment in those days when even using the word was an affectation settled in my prostate and slowly caused some cells to mutate. Diesel fuel aroma, maybe, or fumes off the melted lead pots from which we cast type and made press plates for the newspaper. I inhaled those almost every day for twenty-two years. Or printer's ink mist or traffic exhausts. Or overhead high-tension wires.

But thousands of men who do not have prostate cancer ate as I did and worked as I did. What contrary gene in my anatomy discovered what trigger that fired off my problem?

Science doesn't know. But it has some suspicions. What I, or we, can do about preventing a disease with so many unidentified probable causative factors I can't say. Yet I found investigations into some of the exposures that might—it is still "might"—provoke carcinoma of the prostate so intriguing to me and other victims that they should be a supplemental part of my report to you. Maybe they give us some hints in guiding the habits of our male children, if that is ever possible.

We'll see that as dietary research reports have accumulated over the past several years they've become increasingly positive about the negative effects of animal fats and oils defined as "alpha-linolenic" in our diets, especially as we get older. As far as I know no warnings are posted routinely by our doctors against these possible dangers. Maybe certain foods should have warning labels, like cigarette packages or booze bottles cautioning men susceptible to prostate cancer. This subject, about which researchers have grown less and less tentative in their pronouncements, doesn't seem to have reached even the National Institutes of Health advisory nutrition experts. A 1990 booklet (NIH Publication No. 91-2079) titled "Eating Hints, Tips and Recipes for Better Nutrition during Cancer Treatment" doesn't mention prostate cancer. It presents several recipes suitable for victims in various stages of treatments for other cancers, including radiation, but it doesn't mention that an incipient or potentially recurrent cancer patient should reduce his red meat diet. Details to come.

Are We What We Eat?

Although Dr. Gittes pointed out only a few years ago that no consistent correlation has been found to relate prostate cancer with diet, venereal disease, sexual habits, smoking, or occupational exposure, progressive studies increasingly focus on diet as an important environmental consideration in tumor growth.

The widely varying distribution of prostate cancer in different geographies has strongly suggested that diets, perhaps over a man's lifetime, may cause, prevent, or otherwise influence the development of prostatic cancer. Broadly, parts of the world where fish and vegetables and little of red meats are eaten reflect lower rates than those found in the U.S. and northern Europe where heavier diets prevail.

A group of doctors in Israel closely questioned 964 patients of the Urological Department of the Western Galilee Regional Hospital in Nahariya who had various cancers of the urinary tract; 21.1 percent had cancer of the prostate; 65 percent cancer of the bladder.[3]

Oversimplifying their conclusions, groups that drank the most liquids, consumed the most olive oil and used the most spices, especially cumin, had the lowest incidence of cancers.

I don't care that I already have it: after studying this report I've gone to olive oil for cooking, cumin for spices and more liquids. (Cumin is a spice in general cooking use, mostly in curries.)

Led by Dr. Wilhelm A. Bitterman, the six doctors and one Ph.D. statistician on the team noted that Jews, who made up only 35 percent of the population of their district, had far more prostate cancer than non-Jews, who were 65 percent of the area population. In 1988, 71 percent of the new urologic cancer patients in that region were Jews. The Jews themselves represented two distinct ethnic groups: the Askenazi or European Jews and the Sephardic or Mediterranean-Oriental Jews. The European group, again, had the highest incidence of urologic cancer.

The supply and quality of foodstuffs were identical for all groups. However, the cancer group tended to drink far less fluids in a day than the control groups: most drank ten cups or less per day. Only about a fourth of the control group drank that little; most of those exceeded fifteen cups per day and it seemed to make little difference what the fluids were: coffee, water, tea, fruit juice, or light beverages. Apparently it was the quantity of fluids not the type that was important. The non-Jewish group consumed the highest rate of liquids.

Oils were divided into three groups: (1) olive oil; (2) corn oil, sunflower oil, safflower oil, and some others; and (3) soya, cottonseed, soybean, and some others. Group 3 oils contain alpha-linolenic acid, which also occurs in animal fats. The dominant oil used by the cancer patient group was the soya group. Olive oil, containing both linoleic and linolenic acid, was used predominantly by the non-cancer group which, the study states, may mean that olive oil is good for your genito-urinary system or that the other oils have a negative influence. Olive oil is used most by the non-Jewish population.

Other statistics, which I'll not elaborate, suggested that olive oil, with its unsaturated fatty acids, joins that group of monounsaturated oils that help lower cholesterol levels compared with saturated fats. The team noted reports that Mediterranean populations who consume a lot of olive oil have fewer heart attacks, and so they checked their cardiology records and, sure enough, among their previous two hundred cases of myocardial infarctions in their hospital, 68 percent were Jews and 32 percent non-Jews. This was a fascinating subject but in the scientific world established only that far more study would be required to prove anything substantive. Nevertheless, people have gone on diets with less evidence.

Almost half of the control group used cumin regularly in their diets and two-thirds of them used pepper. The cancer patient group used far less cumin and substantially less pepper. Among the Jewish ethnic groups, fewer Sephardic cancer patients used cumin compared with the Sephardic control groups. Similar ratio with pepper. The scientists determined that cumin inhibits indirectly the formation of "prostaglandin-endoperoxides," bodily chemicals which may act as tumor promoters. I recalled when I saw this report that prostaglandin E1 is one of the drugs that may be injected in the penis to restore erections. The Israeli team didn't get into that subject nor did they relate diet to potency nor open the question of prostaglandin as a possible carcinogen catalyst.

They did further speculate on the low incidence of heart disease in areas where spices are standard portions of regular diets. Tracing the catalytic effect of certain fatty acids in the body, they noted that a digestive enzymatic action takes place that increases the level of a substance called interleukin-2 which may in turn activate the body's natural killer cells. This would increase cytotoxic T-cells (that kill bad cells) and so reduce tumor formation.

Examinations of the interaction of various acids in the human system involve complex reactions which the scientists express in molecular charts and equations that add up to a major academic and medicinal discipline.

This is a lot to lay on fluids, olive oil, cumin, and peppers, but I like spices anyway, never have consumed the standard grammar school mandate of eight glasses of water a day, and while not making a fad out of it, at our house we've been using olive oil as a cooking and salad oil for a couple of years, at least. Since I am in the prostate brotherhood despite that, I must have started too late.

The *Journal of the National Cancer Institute* has published a series of reports on dietary studies based on the hypothesis that food does come into direct contact with many body parts, but conceding that measuring the effects of these contacts is a relatively crude process and the relationships among various dietary components are complex and poorly understood. Unlike most other findings, their 1990 report on a symposium on prostate cancer incidence in the Pacific Basin states and countries found no difference between groups tending toward saturated fat intake and others. They also debated the effect of vitamin A, observing greater dietary risks in the use of vitamin A supplements, not the natural vitamin, and, as a note, not vitamin C supplements. The same report said, in part, "Findings rather consistently showed a positive association with dietary fat intake; however, the data for dietary forms of vitamin A are conflicting."[4]

Another 1990 study suggested protective effects of vitamin A, that perhaps it inhibits cancer progression. It said, "Any factor that hindered this progression would still be important. In a slowly progressive disease like prostate cancer, which has a late clinical onset, inhibition ought to be almost as beneficial as prevention." Yet it quibbled: "Dietary studies appear to be almost evenly divided in suggesting protective or harmful effects of higher intakes of vitamin A, which is usually measured as retinol and B-carotene combined."[5]

Moving toward ever more definitive conclusions, the *Journal of the National Cancer Institute* in October, 1993, published an article, of which Dr. Edward Giovannucci was the lead author, and an editorial by Dr. Kenneth J. Pienta and Peggy S. Esper.[6] The Giovannucci study used data from a Health Professionals questionnaire of 51,529 American men started in 1986 and followed up in 1988 and 1990. The researchers asserted a confidence rank of 95 percent in the results.

Total fat consumption was found directly related to risk of advanced prostate cancer. Red meat represented the food group with the most positive association with advanced cancer. Fat from dairy products (excepting butter) or fish was found unrelated to risk. Saturated fat, monounsaturated fat, and alpha-linolenic acid, but not linolenic acid, were associated with advanced cancer risk. One qualification was that these foodstuffs did not appear to initiate prostate cancer but to elevate the risk of existing, perhaps very early or recurring cancers.

A Pienta-Esper editorial comment on the NCI study said, "The promotion of this disease appears to be linked to an environmental cause, and dietary fat currently seems to be the most likely environmental culprit."

The Giovannucci study suggested strongly that indicators of disease progression, including death, were strongly related to animal fat and that "dietary fat was associated strictly with aggressive cancers." Studying this relationship led to speculation about the interaction of linoleic acids (olive oil, for example) with alpha-linolenic acids (animal fats, for example) that compete in the body for the same digestive enzymes with the result that low levels of linoleic acid (like olive oil) increase the risk of prostate cancer growth.

The following foodstuffs, containing alpha-linolenic acids, were reported to have the most significant associations with advanced prostatic cancer: bacon, butter, mayonnaise, creamy salad dressings, and beef, pork, and lamb as main dishes. Fat from vegetable sources and dairy products, except for butter, were not associated with prostate cancer risk. Other lifestyle items, such as smoking and obesity, were found unrelated to risk of advanced cancers.

Diets high in linoleic acid appear to reduce the risk of cancer progression. Diets high in alpha-linolenic acids may triple the risk of metastasis. In this study, men who ate the most red meat and chicken with skin could face a 3.5 times greater chance of developing an advanced prostate cancer than men in the lower end of the consumption scale.

Just how various foods and their enzymatic competition reach and affect the prostate was not tracked for the lay reader, but it is the result of a chain of interactions involving the complex chemical structures of foods in the digestive process.

Diet as a preventative or a stimulant to prostate cancer makes for challenging speculation, but keep in mind that prostate cancer is not only slow growing but can lie dormant for years, so any dietary cause or protection might have to be traced back over years of consumption. The more recent NCI study of dietary fats did cover protracted eating habits. The study also speculated that since the meat diet was cooked, carcinogens might be formed in the cooking. Many compounds so formed tend to enter and accumulate in the prostatic fluids.

While much of the press I saw—and how much can one person see?—did not cover the Giovannucci report in great detail, it did excerpt the salient points with clarity. Jerry Bishop of the *Wall Street Journal* quoted NCI scientists as emphasizing that the results "should be viewed as tentative and preliminary." I must say they didn't read that way to me given the study's 95 percent level of confidence. Reporter Bishop also gave the meat industry an opportunity for rebuttal. Dr. Eric Hentges of the National Livestock and Meat Board in Chicago said, "How they can make a meat story out of this is beyond me." He termed it a linolenic acid story and said the levels of the acid in soybean oil is seven times higher than in meat. Please recall the Israel hospital report earlier in this chapter in which soybean oil was in group 3, the group of oils most used by the highest prostate cancer cohort of that study.

Jane Brody of the *New York Times* the day after the report was released caught its salient features: heavy meat diets may change prostate cancers from dormancy to possibly lethal malignancy; those who consume an average of 88.6 grams of fat a day have a 79 percent greater chance of developing advanced prostate cancer than those who average 53.2 grams of fat daily.

The *New York Times* report said that Dr. Ernst Wynder, director of the American Health Foundation, proposed a study that would place men with early prostate cancers on a controlled low-fat diet to see if it cut their chances of an advanced or fatal cancer. Reporter Jane E. Brody said the foundation is to start such a study among two thousand women with early stage breast cancer, half of whom would reduce their usual fat intake by more than half, to 15 percent of daily calories.

My studies on this subject left me with the same general advice my mother gave me when I was little: drink lots of fluids, eat plenty of fresh vegetables, and trim the fat off your steaks. I'm going to expand that for myself since my radiation may have missed some lurking microscopic cells. I will rarely enjoy in the future any red meat or chicken-with-skin. Maybe never. Anyway, less than 50 grams.

Environmental Factors

Whether your work environment might encourage prostate cancer troubled several researchers in the past four or five years. In Sweden, doctors checked male nitrate fertilizer workers over a twenty-three-year period and found no association with stomach or prostate cancer, although the incidence of prostate cancer was slightly higher than expected in a normal population cohort.

Cadmium has been suspected for years, and a study by the University of Utah observed a "small increased relative risk" among men working with cadmium compared to other occupational exposures. In passing, this study found statistically more cases among men working in mining, paper and wood industries, medicine, science, entertainment, and recreation; and judged cancers less likely in glass, clay and stone, or rubber, plastics, and synthetics environments.

Men working as janitors and in other building service occupations, said the study, showed an increased relative risk for aggressive tumors. How anyone might utilize such a broad sweep of unspecific information escapes me, but these studies demonstrate the scientific eagerness to identify causes. And I don't want a sad-faced comic coming up to me in some improv laugh shop claiming he wasn't warned that the entertainment industry might add to his risk of prostate cancer.

On the other hand, as we editorial writers like to say, a study in England of cadmium-exposed workers found no increased risk of prostate cancer among them and reported that "in the concentrations encountered it appears unlikely that cadmium acts as a prostatic carcinogen." Few of us are likely to wander into a cadmium environment (such as a storage battery factory) but if you happen to, no need to go around clutching your prostate. The decision is a wash.

Among other occupational groups, large-scale studies showing some increased risk ran the gamut through farmers, mechanics, sheet metal workers, and men in several manufacturing industries. A Finnish study found a significant excess of prostate cancer, over and above what might be expected in the general population, for welders. I'm not sure what this means without exact information on what was being welded, the nature of the fluxes and rods used, etc.

Studies of occupational effects have been inconclusive, such as the ones concerning cadmium. An American Cancer Society pamphlet published in 1988 says men who develop prostate cancer are more likely to be married, to have had more sexual partners than average (while married?), and to have been more sexually active in the ten years prior to their diagnosis. You'll have to check for yourself whether you fit that profile. I do not. I suppose the ACS got this information from surveys and interviews, probably not with patients' wives.

Then I came across a later study that directly contradicts the earlier pamphlet. Other doctors writing for lay audiences have noted that non-malignant problems, such as congestive and irritative prostatitis, may arise from sudden changes in sex patterns, stimulation without orgasm and ejaculation, or holding back ejaculation. Yet no solid evidence whatever proves that these frustrating experiences lead to either prostate enlargement or to cancer of the prostate.

Aging and Possible Effects of Youthful Sex Habits

Aging is certainly part of the process, but age at the time of discovery isn't necessarily the age at which the cancer began. It could have been there a long time. Researchers hedge their own survival figures with reference to "lead time bias," the unknown time the cancer has had to grow before being discovered. Since survival time must be measured from a known date—the date of discovery—that figure is distorted by the unknown factor of the tumor's actual beginning.

Age does relate to changes in endocrine gland functions, namely, again, testosterone production, but scientific proof of a connection does not exist. Prostate cancer occurs in younger men, too. Other studies have examined sexual activity, viral infections, connections with nonmalignant disease of the prostate, frustrated sexual experiences in one's youth (intense build-up of pressure in the semen system with no ejaculation), even tooth decay. Only rarely has prostate cancer been induced in animals experimentally by injecting hormones or carcinogens. The cancer has been found almost accidentally in old rats and has been induced in mice with viral stimulation.

In their book *What Every Man Should Know about His Prostate,* Dr. Monroe Greenberger and co-author Mary-Ellen Siegel, M.S.W., give us straightforward doctor-to-patient talk.[8] Dr. Greenberger and Ms. Siegel suggest indirectly that various irritations of the prostate might induce cancer. Not proven, their counsel is nonetheless interesting. They recommend against taking antihistamines, for instance, because they may cause kidney problems and retention of urine. They postulate that tooth decay may travel to irritate the prostate. This was noteworthy to me, as just a year before my prostate cancer was found, I had completed six months of dental problems and infections, had taken aboard numberless antibiotic tablets and wound up losing my uppers. Could there have been a connection?

Greenberger/Seigel further suspect yeast infections, gonorrhea, or even contaminated swimming pools, which can cause, they say, nonmalignant irritations of the prostate, even chronic prostatitis (inflammation). They think more zinc in the diet might be a preventative.[9]

In their view, sex helps relieve congestive prostatitis and they recommend regular sexual activity as good urological practice. Sex may not prevent cancer but most men will feel that this doctor knows how to make you feel better, sick or not.

When he is sexually aroused, a man's production of fluid in the prostate goes up four to ten times the normal accumulation and the pressure can become quite painful. Neither he nor I dare suggest that men therefore appeal to the partner who has frustrated them for pity, and he merely suggests a prostate massage. Dr. Greenberger believes that the prostate becomes programmed to a certain sexual pace and that delayed ejaculation in either intercourse or masturbation damages the bodily rhythms and can lead to irritation of the gland. He goes into some detail about the efficacy of prostatic massage by a physician. You'll recall Dr. Rous in his book advises against excessive massages.

"Young men need the ejaculatory experience," Greenberger/Siegel write, recalling one patient, however, who suffered reverse problems after (he asserted to the doctor) a marathon indulgence of eleven times in three days. "Feast or famine extremes are not a good idea," said the doctor. He pointed out also that constant vibration, such as when driving a truck, tricks the prostate into thinking something more interesting is going on and can cause excessive fluid production, hence congestion and irritation. He hastens to add, and I emphasize, there is no proven connection between all this and the development of prostate cancer. It may help us understand some of our other genital mysteries, however.

Our Hormones May Hurt Us

Research into hormonal effects may be the most rewarding avenue to finding causes. Men's production of hormones changes with age. Both the testes and the adrenal gland produce testosterone off which the malignant cells "feed."

Black men produce up to 15 percent more testosterone, the male hormone, than whites. Researchers suspect this is one of the reasons blacks develop more and earlier prostate cancer than whites. Others disagree. They blame racial cancer differences on social and economic factors.

The skin and other glands also produce traces of testosterone. Removal or counteraction of testosterone is one of the oldest and most favored treatments, especially in more advanced cases. Prostate cancer is extremely rare in castrated men, for example, and castration, either surgically or through hormonal medication is an accepted treatment for advanced disease, meaning when there is cancer beyond the prostate.

23

The Numbers:
Can We Depend on Them?
Maybe Statistics Hide the Answers

PROSTATE CANCER EMERGED from the closet in the early nineties. Men began to admit to friends and family they had the disease. Prominent show business and political figures went public. Senate Minority Leader Bob Dole (R-Kans.) took up the cudgels for larger research appropriations, noting that federal research dollars for breast cancer exceeded prostate cancer about seven to one. Years of laborious work by statisticians began to pay off in public recognition of the pervasiveness of the illness.

In the accumulation of statistics on discovery, on various treatments and results, and on ages of discovery and of death, perhaps lie some answers to the enigma of this disease. If nothing else, the stats tell the doctors what appears to be working well and what isn't, which therapies are reliable and which aren't. One current debate drawing press attention is whether more early discoveries are worth the trouble, considering the increased number of treatments they'll require. Is this a legitimate argument? Thousands may have cancers so slow growing they will die of something else, never knowing they are ill. Thousands will discover their cancers too late to be cured. Their treatment will be expensive. Discovery is terribly important to the individuals in whom cancer is found, and I think they'll want the searching to continue regardless of cost.

Fernand Labrie, M.D., of Quebec, with his colleagues a cutting-edge pioneer in hormonal treatment research, estimated that seventy-five million men now alive in the world have or will have a prostate cancer serious enough to require treatment.[1]

In each decade of man's life after forty, his chance of getting prostate cancer will double. In the past few years it has exceeded lung cancer as a killer, about 38,000 men a year. Some 165,000 cases were reported in 1993 and 200,000 are expected in 1994, with increased screening accelerating those figures through the decade. In the past, anywhere from a fourth to a third of the number of new cases later became statistics for deaths from prostate cancer. Deaths reported were not new cases, of course. Death figures were of victims counted among new cases perhaps two to twenty years ago.

The Cancer Statistics Review of the National Cancer Institute shows a rate of prostate cancer for black males at 132 per 100,000 and for white males at 88 per 100,000. The average annual death rate from prostate cancer is given at 23.4 per 100,000. The doctor-statisticians expect the number of cases to explode as we approach the next century because of growth in the aged population, better discovery techniques, and improved awareness among men at risk.

Prostate cancer victims form a sizeable brotherhood. Juggling the figures a little, I'd estimate there are at this minute from 750,000 to a million men alive today in the United States who during the past decade were diagnosed with prostate cancer and that upwards of another 250,000 to 300,000 have died of prostate cancer during those ten years.

This is a statistics-prone field. Accumulated statistics help guide physicians in their treatment options and increase their ability to discuss with a patient his probable futures.

In my studies for this book, I learned also not to take too literally statistics regarding mortality, longevity after the discovery of a cancer, the comparative benefits of various treatments, and the efficacy of assorted diagnostic procedures. Your urologist does considerable reading; he is equipped to evaluate each reported study and statistical bank as it appears, but the layman is not. One must absorb a continuing flow of statistics, tempered by experience, in order to base a course of medical action upon them.

The size of the study population, the patients' ages, and the range of cancer involvement when discovered in patients (whether confined to the prostate or spread) forces research into several discrete categories. Even the matter of categorizing a patient's prostate cancer in order to determine treatment is itself a subject of continuing study and debate among physicians and is not as precise as they would like. For instance, a study of less than a few hundred patients results in imprecise percentages of survival, regression, effective treatments, and so forth. A study of one hundred patients over a period of several years may result in a five-year survival rate (after treatment) for a categorical subgroup of twenty-five. With such a small base, one patient's survival or death could change the percentages not by 4 percent but by 8 percent, because the patient adds to one column and deducts from another.

Statistics are also affected if some men in these studies die of causes other than prostate cancer, from heart attacks to traffic accidents, and so dilute the precision of the reports. If you see statistical reports on your own, such as the monthly reports from the National Cancer Institute, you'll be less frightened if you maintain a sense of perspective about them.

Statistics for small studies don't always agree with the percentages from larger studies. Data bases vary. Official statistics are issued by the American Cancer Society (ACS), the National Cancer Institute (NCI), and something called SEER, established by Congress in the National Cancer Act of 1971. SEER stands for Surveillance, Epidemiology, and End Results. The SEER covers an estimated 9.6 percent of the U.S. population and its data base, tracking all forms of cancer, includes more than 1.5 million cases. SEER gets reports from hospitals, abstracts of death certificates on which cancer is listed as a cause in the records of diagnostic clinics, radiotherapy units, and other central information sources.

As a case in point, the five- and ten-year survival rates for prostate cancer victims in discrete categories reported herein derive from a base of 81,950 cases between 1974 and 1986. A new world of prostate cancer has emerged since 1986. Reports from more recent studies are so noted. But you can't get an early 1990s figure for ten-year survival unless you start counting from diagnoses in the early 1980s.

Somewhat conflicting statistics say that from one in eight to one in eleven men will have this tumor. About 80 percent of all prostate cancers will be diagnosed in men sixty-five or older, and the average age of discovery is seventy-three. Less than 1 percent of clinically detectable prostate cancers occur in men under fifty, but the younger the victim the more dangerous the tumor.

Black Americans have the highest incidence and Japanese Americans the lowest. Blacks produce up to about 15 percent more testosterone, the male hormone, than whites, and since cancer cells respond to testosterone that is suspected but not proven as a cause. The higher mortality among blacks has been blamed also in part on late diagnosis, a result of widespread economic deprivation, and lack of information.

Ruben Gittes, M.D., in the *New England Journal of Medicine* (Jan. 1991), speculates that since latent cancer found in autopsies is about the same for all ethnic and racial groups, a direct genetic cause is unlikely. However, he goes on to report that men who have both an affected first-degree relative (a brother or father) and an affected second-degree relative (an uncle or grandfather) have an eightfold increase in risk. So testosterone and diets relatively high in red meats and low in vegetables, combined with race, may predict the incidence of prostate cancer in various groups, Dr. Gittes says, adding that the hypothesis needs further testing.

Since his report, it has been tested in several studies with blame being placed more and more on fatty diets. (See chap. 22.)

Another leading researcher and physician, in a more recent study, maintains the black-white numbers are a statistical anomaly and that if there is a difference in racial vulnerability, it is because blacks present with the disease some five years earlier in life than whites and in general eat foods high in fat.

Benign but serious ailments of the prostate will affect many millions more. A Harvard report says that 350,000 prostate resections (TURPs) will be performed each year to relieve symptoms of enlarged prostates. About 10 to 20 percent of these may reveal concealed cancer when tissues from the operation are analyzed. I have no new figure, but changing methods of treating BPH (benign prostatic hyperplasia) are substituting for TURPs, perhaps reducing the TURP incidence as much as a third.

It is not that figures lie and liars figure. It is that only fairly large studies produce reliable percentages, and even in these, the definitions and classifications of data must be reported with finite accuracy. Maintaining and interpreting data from dozens of sources on thousands of cases, which may not have been accurately classified (according to stages, grades, ages of men, presence of other diseases, workplaces, diets, early histories of disease, dental problems, etc.) not only is difficult but expensive.

Discuss it with your congressperson. Part of the answer is money.

24

Reference

The TNM Staging System, and Some Others

WE EXAMINED "STAGING" routines in part 1 and displayed one of the most frequently used, the ABCD system.

Another system you should be aware of (I'm not going to list all of them) has come into more recent use and professional publications have started using it instead of the ABCD system. This is the TNM method, and you may come across it frequently in your prostate cancer reading. You may see both systems used together for clarity. (Incidentally, the American Cancer Society publishes a card guide to all tumor classifications.)

TUMOR

TX—the primary tumor cannot be assessed

T0—no evidence of primary tumor

T1—clinically inapparent tumor, not palpable, not visible by imaging;

    T1a: incidental cells found in 5 percent or less of tissue analyzed

    T1b: incidental cells found in more than 5 percent of tissue

    T1c: tumor identified by needle biopsy (because of PSA elevation)

T2—tumor confined within prostate

    T2a: tumor involves half of a lobe or less

    T2b: tumor involves more than half a lobe but not both sides

    T2c: tumor involves both lobes

T3—tumor extends through the prostatic capsule

    T3a: extracapsular extension one side (unilateral)

    T3b: extracapsular extension both sides (bilateral)

    T3c: tumor invades seminal vesicle(s)

T4—tumor is fixed or invades adjacent structures other than seminal vesicles

    T4a: tumor invades any of the following: bladder neck, external sphincter, rectum

    T4b: tumor invades muscles and/or is fixed to pelvic wall

REGIONAL LYMPH NODE INVASION

NX—regional lymph nodes cannot be assessed

N0—no regional node metastasis

N1—metastasis in a single lymph node, 2cm or less

N2—metastasis in a single node, more than 2cm but not more than 5cm

N3—metastasis in a node more than 5 cm

DISTANT METASTASIS

MX—presence of metastasis cannot be assessed

M0—no distant metastasis

M1—distant metastasis

    M1a: nonregional lymph node(s)

    M1b: metastasis in bone(s)

    M1c: metastasis in other site(s)

When metastasis is present in more than one site, the most advanced category is used which would be M1c.

This TNM system is somewhat more specific than the A–D system in sizing the tumors and locating them more precisely. It is useful in research and in comparing treatment results. You may run across it in your reading.

As an example, you might see this phrase: T1N0M0. That would mean a tumor the urologist could not feel with his finger, and is within the normal prostate capsule with no lymph node involvement and no metastasis evident.

There is also a "Hopkins" system that incorporates microscopic findings according to the percentage of tissue examined. There is a Stanford system that goes like this:

T0—occult carcinoma, present but not active

T1—palpable tumor limited to the prostate without distortion of the boundaries

T2—palpable tumor limited to the prostate with minimal distortion of the boundaries

T3—palpable tumor extending beyond the capsule obliterating portions of adjacent tissues or of the seminal vesicle region

T4—palpable tumor extending beyond the capsule with attachment to the pelvic side wall or rectal or bladder invasion

Staging-Related Procedures

Common procedure in the immediate past has been that lymph node biopsies will not be made on a patient who is to be treated with radiation, while it is standard procedure for a surgeon performing a radical prostatectomy to analyze lymph nodes as he starts the surgical procedure. So surgeons discover understaging more definitively than do radiologists, since the practice has been not to expose the patient to surgery in order to obtain lymph node tissue. With the advent of laparoscopy, an easier and less traumatic way to access the nodes, more radiation patients will receive a lymph node examination. Dr. Nash is setting a laparoscopic lymphade-nectomy (removal of lymph node tissues) as a standard if he is suspicious of spread. Tumor in the lymph nodes means a D1 cancer, at best. It is this discovery as well as others during surgery that frequently prove that the stage initially assigned was an underestimate. It is the pathology lab's ex-amination of the removed prostate that ultimately tells this story, so under-staging of many radiation patients may never be definitively discovered.

One recent intensive conference on staging resulted in several recom-mendations from what impressed me as a pretty sharp crowd of medics focused on their patients' interests. How they would implement their ideas I'm not sure and neither were they, but basically they want uniformity in evaluating and diagnosing prostate cancer. One doctor said during the meeting that it became clear to him that the ability to evaluate various treat-ment methods is seriously limited because different grading systems are used and meaningful comparisons are compromised or negated if patient groups have been stratified differently.

This conference report even urged that the editorial policies of the major journals in urology and pathology should try to achieve this kind of uniformity so everyone knows precisely what everyone else is talking about. "To date," one doctor said, "a clear concensus has not been reached re-garding which of over forty grading systems published in the literature should be uniformly adopted."

Dr. Donald Coffey, Ph.D., a professor of urology at Johns Hopkins who is originally from Tennessee, insists at conferences and in his lectures that new methods of analyzing and fighting prostate cancer must be found. However, the good professor also manages to inject a little levity into oth-erwise stultifyingly sober meetings. For example, at one meeting he sug-gested this "Tennessee" staging system:

Stage 1	Tetched
Stage 2	Right Much
Stage 3	Et up
Stage 4	Plum et up
Stage 5	Daid

25

The Doctor's TURP Strategy
What's on His Mind While He's "In There"?

CAN WE KNOW MORE about prostate cancer and the various ministrations employed in its treatment than is good for us? Should we know only what "they" tell us? I've had brethren of the prostate tell me, "I don't want to know that much about it. I've got enough on my mind." I'm at the other extreme. I want to know all about it, including what the surgeon's thinking while he's chiseling out part of my gland. For those with a similar level of curiosity, this chapter expands on the chapter in part 1 titled "The Turrible Turp." You'll probably get well just as fast without it, but you may also find it interesting.

*   *   *

When Cy Nash and I were discussing the precise surgery used in excavating (not a medical term) an enlarged prostate to relieve BPH (benign prostatic hyperplasia) I asked him to review the mental strategies exercised as he prepares for the transurethral resection.

He said, "With any operation you have to approach it this way: how am I going to get into trouble? It's just like anything else. You know when you fly—anybody could fly—but you think to yourself, how am I going to screw up and crash? What's going to happen? What are the three, four, five, six things that are going to make this thing a failure?

"The balloon's got to be in the right place, otherwise the man can be incontinent. All the chips have to be out, otherwise the catheter's going to plug and you'll have to change the catheter and the patient's going to bleed more. And every time you manipulate it the patient can get septic, infected. You have to stop the bleeding. You can't overload his system with fluid. If you have a patient who comes to the operating room in a little congestive failure, you better dry him out first because you're going to give him more fluid through his vessels.

"So all these things have to be just right to have a good operation, to have good success. Now. If the operating doctor coagulates too much over here, or over here, he could damage the sphincter. Or if he cuts too far back, he could damage the sphincter. Then the patient could be incontinent. It's just like anything else. You have to know how you get into trouble, and to avoid those situations and to get your technique down right. You're thinking, how you are going to get into trouble; the rest of the stuff anybody could do."

I recalled that all the cutting, coagulation, and maneuvering takes place in the interior of an organ no bigger than a walnut. That "anybody" could do it, I doubted.

He caught my expression. "Well, this is an unusual operation. You assume every surgeon knows how to do an appendix or a hernia, right? But not every urologist knows how to do a good TURP. Some just make a tunnel, perhaps take out an adequate amount for that particular patient although a tunnel is not a complete TURP; some go too deep, some get too much bleeding, because everyone has his own level of skill. Some urologists don't like to do them, some do too many.

"If the surgeon hasn't had good experience with a larger than usual gland, he should do a cut—an open subtotal prostatectomy. For example, Dr. A may do a 50 gram prostate very nicely but if he gets to 80 grams, he's lost, gets bad results, so Dr. A if it's 80 grams will make an open incision to take out that prostate enlargement.

"This is not a cancer operation I'm talking about. This is just to take out the fruit. The prostate, say, is like an orange. You take out the fruit and you have a shell left. When you do radical surgery you take the whole thing out. In other words, if you are doing a TURP you want to get all this tissue out and just leave this capsule's rim of tissue, so that you have a big cavity in there. Some people just make a little tunnel, some people take out more.

"If you go through the capsule and perforate it, you could get extravasation of fluid [*permitting fluid to leak*], so it's a very technical operation. This tissue could be removed through the penis or by cutting into the bladder or by cutting into here [*gestures just above the pubic area*] and you cut it out and you leave the shell. When you have a cancer you have to take out everything, the capsule, the gland itself, the seminal vesicle alongside the gland. But what we're talking about now is removing prostatic tissue to relive pressure on the urethra. Now, your question is, when do you stop removing tissue in doing a TURP? The capsule, or shell, looks different than prostate tissue. When you've finished with the "fruit," you see the different tissue of the shell and you stop."

Are these techniques and the tools inserted through the penis new developments?

Cy said, "The method of using an electric loop for cutting and coagulation has been around a long time, maybe sixty years. We've had several modifications but the basic elements are the same.

"Inserting a lamp so we can see in there with the resectoscope started longer ago, something like 1920. We didn't have fiber optics then, of course. We used to use a tiny flashlight hooked up to an electric battery and the light would go in with its wire. Fiber optics is a lot better.

"There's another operational instrument available that captures the fluid as it comes out. It is an Iglesias modification of the Iglesias resectoscope. Iglesias was a Cuban urologist who came here to Miami after Castro. He lived on the Beach (the city of Miami Beach) for a while. He invented a lot of instruments. He moved to Newark, N.J., and was in a department of the New Jersey State Medical School at Newark. He developed a new device where the fluid can go in and you can have suction available, too. We sometimes need the suction to make sure all the pieces are out. It saves time. The surgeon doesn't have to stand up and empty the bladder all the time. The process is called continuous irrigation."

Possible problems with irrigating fluids and solutions alarmed me. They don't tell you that stuff before they operate.

"That's basic information," Cy said. "We learn that early. Every now and then an inexperienced nurse may put up saline by mistake. That would disperse the electric current you need. You just look at the bag and say, 'What the hell did you do this for?' So we have a sign in that room that only glycine is supposed to be put up there.

"Now, in addition to that, the fluid is absorbed by the body. You're cutting open vessels and that speeds up the absorption. If that fluid is water, your patients could get a severe hemolytic anemia [*red blood cells can absorb too much water and be destroyed*]. Early on, there were a number of deaths from this operation because patients were absorbing too much water, and dying. So, your solution has to be nonelectrolytic and nonhemolytic, so the blood cells won't absorb it. That's where the sugars come in.

"About fifty years ago they realized they had to use something other than water or saline solution. If you resected and you had a lot of vessels open, the patient could absorb this fluid and get water intoxication—that's even with the right solution—so if you operate too long and too many vessels are open, too much fluid is absorbed; it dilutes the patient's serum sodium [*blood salt level*] and he could become hyponatremic [*low blood sodium*], and suffer water intoxication."

The plaster model Dr. Nash used to illustrate his points included the lower portion of the bladder. "Yes," he responded to my gesture. "We go into the bladder. Anyway, the cystoscope will go into the bladder and look around the bladder. The resectoscope can go anywhere in there because if there is a bladder tumor here or there, the same instrument that I do the prostate with I use to resect the bladder cancer. So this instrument can go there and if the patient has a very long penis or is very big, we have bigger instruments."

I said, "OK. I also know you are working hard to prevent infection during surgery. What do you do with those who have infections before surgery?"

"Certainly if the patient's had infected urine beforehand, we try to clear that up, and we would never operate on someone who had acute epididymitis or prostatitis or anything like that. If my patients come in with such a problem, I treat them and send them home. You don't operate in the face of those problems."

"Cy, you seem to concentrate especially on controlling bleeding after the operation."

"That's right. We want the blood to come out around the catheter. Then the urine, going through the catheter, may be perfectly clear. Most of the bleeders are at the bladder neck. The irrigating fluid goes in and comes out as it should, through the catheter."

"Isn't the catheter balloon preventing blood flowing out?"

"No. Beyond the apex of the prostate is the external sphincter. If this balloon is not blown up enough and it goes into this cavity then it lies on the sphincter and we don't want that. So you have to make sure the balloon is in the right place, that there's the right pressure, not too tight; you must make sure that the catheter doesn't get blocked with blood clots, that's why we have the continuous irrigation and we must make sure that all the chips we cut out are gone, because that one chip can block that catheter and then if there's no outflow and there's continued inflow, the patient's bladder will enlarge, he will have a lot of pain and you will have to change the catheter and every time you change the catheter you stir up the bleeding again. So the trick that enables me to sleep well at night and not have to run back to the hospital is to make sure all of these things that I mentioned are done properly.

Sometimes if there's bleeding we add certain drugs that will help, like Amicar, either by mouth or intravenously, to stop the bleeding, because after prostatic surgery there's an increase in what we call urokinase which lyses [*dissolves*] blood clots. The Amicar blocks this process, because we want the little vessels to clot and not lyse."

"Urokinase? Is that an enzyme?" I may have been showing off a little.

"Yes, that's a bodily enzyme. It is part of a natural process that goes on in the body all the time. When a blood clot forms in the coronary arteries, the patient is given streptokinase into the heart, into the coronary blood vessels, to lyse or dissolve the clot and prevent heart muscle damage. There's a new drug that costs $2,000. The streptokinase costs $200. There was a study concerning the old stuff that's been around twenty-five or thirty years and it turned out the streptokinase was just as good as this new biologically made TPA that cost $2000 a shot, so a new treatment may be a fad but it's not always the best. The urokinase is like streptokinase only they call it urokinase because it lyses the clots in the urine. So we block that with Amicar, because we don't want the clots to lyse, we want clotting to occur in the blood vessels so that the bleeding will stop."

"What about some of the new procedures, such as the balloon to dilate a partially blocked urethra?" I asked.

"It's experimental. It's for people with only certain types of prostate glands. It's not for people who have cancer of the prostate. If your prostate is too big or you have a large middle lobe, the results are poor.

"With BPH, if you have a young person and the gland is not too big, say a 30 to 40 gram gland, and the patient still wants to have children and so needs to avoid retrograde ejaculation, then it may be justified for him. He may have to have the treatment every two or three years. The balloon dilation is a whole new thing, a separate topic. Actually, the first guys who did the balloons were the radiologists who used the balloons on vessels in the legs or the coronary arteries. They said, why don't we do it for the prostate? A fellow named Castenada from Minnesota began it. It is not going to replace a TURP. A TURP is the 'gold standard' for treating this problem."

"At one point, you said you 'stand up.' Do you do this operation sitting down?" I asked.

"I sit down most of the time but there are times when I go like this, or like that [*he bobs and weaves like a basketball player*] to see what I need to see through the scope. I am standing when the fluid comes out, usually, and when I'm cutting I'm usually sitting, or I may be standing. My anterior thigh muscles are good because I may stand for an hour going like this and it takes good muscles. If you've got poor muscles, or a bad neck or back, you can't do a good TURP because physically a good TURP can be a real workout . . . it's good for my tennis, too. Really, I'm like this [*crouching, standing, etc.; remember, he is moving a light inside the prostate while keeping his eye glued to the lens of the resectoscope*], dipping down, like hitting a tennis ball.

"I suppose you could say urologists face an occupational hazard. They can get cervical disk problems, arthritis, or spinal cord pressure doing TURPs. A colleague of mine recently had to undergo a cervical laminectomy [*removal of the bony covering of areas of the spine*] to relieve pressure on his cervical spinal cord."

"Let me ask a patient question instead of a reporter question. Why do you think the TURP was needed before I start radiation therapy?"

"Some patients get into trouble with radiation if they have symptoms because they're not emptying their bladder, or if they have urgency or excessive frequency in urination then," he said. "If we irradiate in the face of those symptoms, or, say, before doing a TURP, these symptoms may be aggravated. The patient can go into retention and require a catheter. Radiation for the cancer is then not as effective, or the radiation may have to be stopped and later restarted, which means poorer results. That's why I did the TURP on you first. I had a half dozen patients in the past year or two that I treated the same way and they breezed through the radiation. The patients who have a lot of trouble are those who needed something done even before the radiation, because of obstructions."

26

The PSA Revolution

How PSA and Ultrasound Changed the Landscape

IN APRIL, 1991, the *New England Journal of Medicine* published a report by Dr. William Catalona and several of his associates at the Washington University School of Medicine and Barnes Hospital in St. Louis, Mo., on PSA as a screening test for prostate cancer.

Dr. Catalona's article triggered considerable ink and pictures in the public press and on television, where PSA was treated as a new and dramatic discovery related to prostate cancer. It was that, but unfortunately, from many of the stories that resulted, the reader or viewer might believe PSA amount to a cure and that it had just been identified.

Drs. G. P. Murphy, M. C. Wang, and L. A. Valenzuela opened the way to PSA analysis in 1979 when they published their discovery and isolation of the specific glycoprotein produced by the troubled prostate. They were honored for this in 1993. The actual test was first developed in the late seventies by Drs. Thomas Stamey and N. Yang of Stanford who had been searching for a "marker" unique to the prostate. The earliest "immunoassay," the testing kit for measuring prostate specific antigen, bears Dr. Yang's name. Dr. Murphy is a former chief of medicine for the American Cancer Society and is now with the Northwest Tumor Institute in Seattle.

By now, several assays have come on the scene. They are subject to minor differences so you should try to see that the same one is used in any series of tests.

My fellow journalists may have exaggerated somewhat the role of PSA in today's medical environment. However, I join them in regarding the PSA as an exciting new advance, finally being recognized by the medical community for its contribution to prostate cancer discovery and, perhaps as important, as a sensitive measurement of the progression of cancer and its response to treatment. Doctors writing for doctors appear to maintain eminently conservative positions and to curb their enthusiasms. Dr. Catalona favors cautious phrasing, but his confidence in projecting his research findings must have come through to the reporters who based their stories on them. He has adamantly insisted the PSA test scores between 4 and 10, though these figures may often indicate BPH as well, deserve further examinations, including biopsies. About 27 percent of the men with such a reading will have prostate cancer.

Dr. Peter Scardino of Houston wrote in *A.U.A. Today*, September 1991, that with B stage cancers an average of 18 percent will have seminal vesicle invasion and 30 percent will have cancer in the lymph nodes that drain the prostatic region. Dr. Stamey reported he found that with PSA's of 4 to 10, 24 percent of the men examined had prostate cancer, 96 percent of them localized. If the PSA was greater than 10, 65 percent had prostate cancer and only 8 percent were still confined to the capsule.

Well-advanced cancers can produce PSA readings in the thousands. However, poorly differentiated or high Gleason tumors might produce less PSA than would be expected, so a cancer could be worsening and PSA wouldn't track it.

PSA as a Screening Method

At least two teams of doctors, who don't agree precisely with each other on what the numbers mean, now advocate broad population screening using the PSA as an initial test. To evaluate screening usefulness in detection and staging, Dr. Catalona and his associates measured PSA levels in 1,653 healthy men fifty years old or older. Those with PSA values equal to or greater than 4.0 ng/ml were given rectal exams and ultrasound testing, with ultrasound-directed biopsies on those with abnormal readings. They compared these results with tests performed on three hundred men of the same age range who underwent tests because of symptoms or DRE indications. In his April 1991 article, Dr. Catalona wrote:

> From 30 to 50 percent of patients with benign prostatic hyperplasia (BPH) have elevated serum PSA concentrations depending on the size of the prostate and the degree of obstruction, and the concentrations are increased in 25 to 92 percent of patients with prostate cancer, depending on tumor volume. [The percentage range arises from different brackets of the study.] Measurement of serum PSA is the most sensitive marker available for monitoring the progression of prostate cancer and its response to therapy, but its value for the early detection and staging of prostate cancer is not known.

Perhaps Dr. Catalona should have said "not established," because PSA is used widely in staging decisions since it usually relates directly to the volume of tumor present. In the Catalona study, 21 percent of the men with cancer had normal PSA levels. However, for something to be "known" or "established" in the medical world takes a lot more proof than PSA has had time to develop in the six or seven years it has been in general application. Indeed, the landmark article concluded that a combination of PSA and rectal exams, with ultrasonography, provides a better method of detecting prostate cancer than rectal examination alone. I should add that since he wrote this article, Dr. Catalona has strengthened his confidence in the PSA and has devoted a lot of time to refining what it means in each gradation of numbers.

About 65 percent of prostate cancers appear to be localized at the time of diagnosis, Dr. Catalona continues, but only about half of these prove to be confined to the prostate at the time of surgery. This means almost two-thirds, or 65+ percent, have spread beyond the prostate when first identified. A substantial number of cancers can not be felt in a DRE and will be missed by ultrasound, although it is fair to say that some of those missed may be so small as to be insignificant—at that time. In any event, early detection is critical because prostate cancers confined to the gland can be cured. (I know I keep saying this. I'm reminding men to be examined. "Watch and wait" is not for younger men who want to be cured.)

Until recently, the medical fraternity agreed that PSA was not a staging tool. Now, there's a mind shift in progress, as reading it becomes more sophisticated. Increasing understanding of PSA density (PSAD), the relative weight of the prostate to the PSA reading, improves interpretation. Also relatively new is the determination of PSA velocity, its rate of change from time to time, in reading more precisely what the test tells us.

Dr. Stamey reported in a 1989 monograph written for physicians' information that a gram of prostate cancer elevates the serum PSA level at least 10 times as much a gram of BPH.[1] So, if PSA is not a staging tool, it is a major screening one, and its range will have weight in the staging decision. In the Catalona study, for example, all men with 10 ng/ml readings or greater, verified by a second sample, had abnormal or suspicious rectal and/or ultrasonograph readings. Of 107 men with PSA's from 4 to 9.9, 22 percent were found to have prostate cancer. Of 85 men with PSA counts of 10 or more, 67 percent biopsied positively for cancer. I am not going to submerge you with statistics, so, in summary, Dr. Catalona concluded that "serum PSA results provided diagnostic information superior to that provided by age and the two other procedures," that is, DRE (digital rectal exam) and ultrasound.

In the *Journal of Urology*, March 1992 (an entire issue devoted to prostate cancer), Dr. Patrick C. Walsh of Johns Hopkins distinguished some "facts" about prostate cancer from some "true facts." One alleged fact is

that if prostate cancer is detected before it has metastasized and is left untreated, it usually takes longer than ten years to kill the patient. Unfortunately, as Dr. Walsh translated the "true fact," today's methods can't
detect microscopic foci of tumor. So no one really knows exactly when the
cancer began. *So when do we start counting the ten years?* Heed well this re-
spected researcher and surgeon:

> transrectal ultrasonography can miss half of nonpalpable cancers
> greater than 1 cm in size. Each gram of prostate cancer increases se-
> rum prostate specific antigen (PSA) by an average of 3.5 ng/ml [na-
> nograms per milliliter] using the Yang technique, which is 2.3 ng/ml
> with the Hybritech assay. Thus using either technique one is not
> going to be able to detect microscopic foci of cancer. Furthermore, to
> detect a microscopic focus of prostate cancer in a 40 gram prostate,
> one would have to perform more than 100 random needle biopsies
> . . . it should be recognized that today we are diagnosing prostate
> cancer too late, not too early. In carefully selected studies 40 percent
> of the men who undergo radical prostatectomy have extraprostatic
> disease. We need to do a better job.

Walsh continues, pointing out also that many men with prostate cancer
have a PSA of less than 2.8 ng/ml and in the 4 to 10 range benign prostatic
hyperplasia (BPH) confuses the picture. Therefore, he reminds his colleagues, yearly measurements provide greater specificity when PSA elevations are discovered. This is similar to the established practice in breast
cancer where after forty, women are advised to undergo regular mam-
mographies, procedures twice as costly as PSA tests.

Many variables can affect PSA levels. About 20 percent of patients
with enlarged prostates (BPH) have levels exceeding 4 ng/ml. Also some
10 percent of patients with BPH will be found to also have cancer.

An updated study of what might affect a PSA reading also appeared in
the *Journal of Urology,* March 1992, by Dr. Jerry J. J. Yuan and six colleagues, one of whom was Dr. Catalona. All are associated with the Washington School of Medicine in St. Louis. Although they emphasized the
value of taking PSA blood samples prior to any manipulation of the prostate, they found that DRE's, prostatic massage, and ultrasonography had
little effect but that prostatic needle biopsies caused marked elevations in
PSA. They could not prove Dr. Stamey's contention that prostatic massages increased PSA counts twofold, but said the type of assay and the
vigor of the massage may have affected the readings. What did Dr. Nash
tell us? "Nothing in prostate cancer is 100 percent."

Two other studies are reported in that issue of the *Journal of Urology,* by a team from the J. Bentley Squier Urologic Clinic at Columbia University College of Physicians and Surgeons, New York, joined by Dr. William H. Cooner of the University of South Alabama, Mobile, now at Emory University in Atlanta. No urologist would object if I refer to Dr. Cooner as one of the major "deans" of the urologic community.

Let's recall that the tricky area of PSA interpretation lies generally in readings between 4.0 and 10.0. It is in this region that cancer will be found in only about 22 percent of the cases. Checking PSA density (PSAD) is one technique for sharpening diagnoses when the PSA is in this range. PSAD is derived by dividing the ng/ml PSA reading by the weight of the entire prostate. The PSAD number for BPH alone is consistently and significantly lower than the PSAD number when cancer is present. In fact, the risk of cancer increases in direct proportion to increases in PSAD. This makes PSAD invaluable in that indeterminate range between 4 and 10 ng/ml. The researchers are working on a method to find prostate volume with ultrasound, which would be easier and cheaper than with MRI.

There are a couple of major steps forward implicit in PSAD findings. One is that patients within PSA ranges that could mean BPH can be identified as requiring especially aggressive examinations for cancer. The other is that sometimes patients may have a serious cancer and still show a normal PSA. If these men can be identified, they will have a better chance of effective treatment.

Research continues to provide better definitions for PSA. Earlier (in chapter 7) we reported a new scale for minimum readings of PSA that suggest the presence of cancer. A 4.0 ng/ml reading has been the generally accepted level below which a man is considered free of cancer. The newer scale relates PSA to age, so a younger man with a PSA as low as 3.5 would be more closely assessed and a man in his sixties might be cleared of cancer suspicion at 4.5 and one who was seventy or older at 6.5.

A major question in diagnosis concerns identifying nonpalpable (can't feel them) A1 and A2 cancers, distinguishing them from BPH and determining whether they need treatment. In the not too distant past, operations for BPH would produce tissue that could be analyzed and many cancers were located that way. More and more BPH is being treated with medication, lasers, sound waves, and other methods that produce no tissue for the microscopes. As a compensation, perhaps, for the declining use of the TURP, PSA and ultrasound-guided biopsies became more specifically analytical. Thus, for instance, stage A cancers frequently can be classified without the invasive surgery of a TURP. The other side of that coin is that some of the noninvasive methods may affect PSA readings and after treatment the patient's PSA may not be reliable for fine and detailed follow-up interpretation.[2]

One way to get around these constraints is by examining "relative nuclear roundness," the shape of the heart of the cell itself. In A1 and A2 cancers an assessment of whether the cancer will progress can be derived from measuring mean absolute cellular roundness. Of men with A2 cancer it is estimated only 35 percent eventually will die of the disease. The other 65 percent might be spared unnecessary treatment if they could be identified. Measuring "roundness" is time-consuming and tedious.

As you saw in our discussion of the "watch and wait" attitude, especially on A1 cancers that may never develop dangerously, the treatment decision may come down to how to tell which will become threatening. This question has become so alive that some researchers think entirely new staging categories should be devised for them.

Another way to make use of the PSA is to measure its "doubling time." This measurement has been applied primarily in estimating the time to clinical failure after external beam radiation treatment. By identifying a biologically aggressive tumor, it would tell us whether a man with a rising PSA required immediate secondary treatment or could wait for clinical signs of recurring disease. Researchers know that a rising PSA after radiation or a detectable PSA after surgery almost always means recurrent or persistent disease.

The authors of one report correlated the time for the PSA to double (PSA-DT, meaning PSA doubling time) with the time for clinical relapse after failure of an initial procedure showed up in the PSA count.[3] A doubling time of 3.8 months or less, they said, indicates immediate further treatment is needed. If the doubling time is greater than 3.8 months the tumor biology may be far less aggressive and the patient could be spared the cost and side effects of further treatment until the cancer manifested itself clinically. With a PSA doubling time of 18 months or more, the patients might be regularly observed and not treated because "the disease might not become clinically apparent during the patient's lifetime." Of course, the physician has to know when to start the timing.

This knowledge could spare the patient a salvage therapy and, checking against actuarial tables, could mean he might well die of something else before the cancer grew to a point that required treatment. However, the PSA doubling time interpretation is not quite so simple and direct as that, since the disease-free intervals and pretreatment PSA measurements are involved. We do not have to do the calculation, though. All we need to know is that yet another factor in the complex calculus of disease progression seems, when further verified, to give us ever more specific information as to what's going on "down there."

Understanding Ultrasound

At a symposium in Chicago in September 1990, Fred Lee, M.D., reported for a group of doctors from St. Joseph Mercy Hospital in Ann Arbor, Mich., on the use of ultrasound in diagnosis and staging of prostatic carcinoma. Dr. Lee cited progress in the use of ultrasound imaging, with a particular leap forward in 1986 with the development of 7.0 MHz scanning equipment. His group's report takes on the technology in too much detail for our mission here, but it involves the anatomical division of the prostate into distinct zones, how a cancer may travel from zone to zone or into the seminal vesicles, and how ultrasound can guide a biopsy needle more accurately.

"We now understand," the group reports, "areas of anatomical weakness through which the cancer can escape the confines of the prostate. [It escapes through the places where nerves and blood vessels enter the prostate and other weaker areas of the gland that join, or connect with ducts, various other glands.] The role of biopsy has been extended from its use in diagnosis . . . to include evaluation of tumor extension for staging." Drs. Stamey and McNeal of Stanford also have reported major research on this subject.

The Lee group recommended that TRUS (Transrectal UltraSound) guided biopsies be performed first on all palpable lesions. They said, "Studies have shown that up to 50 percent of negative biopsies guided by palpitation [the finger only] have been subsequently proved positive for cancer with TRUS guided biopsy."

In cases where no cancer can be felt in a DRE but is suspected, perhaps because of symptoms or an elevated PSA reading, ultrasound may locate the tumor. If it cannot and the urologist remains suspicious, random biopsies may be made in which the needle scans the prostate in a pattern that should hit a tumor if one is present. Before ultrasound, needle biopsies were done through the rectum or through the crotch behind the scrotum (the perineal area). The patient was anesthetized. A special "gun" developed in Sweden changed that in the late 1980s. The gun is part of the sonogram probe implements inserted in the rectum and fires a thin needle so fast the patient feels no pain, nothing more than a little thump. The ease of the procedure and the accuracy of ultrasound have improved diagnosis and staging.

Because the inserted ultrasound equipment is closer to the prostate than a CT it can "focus" somewhat better. It does have some limitations. Its quality depends considerably on the ability of the examiner and the equipment used. Terms describing what it reads are "echoic," meaning that an area shows the same density as the surrounding tissue in the prostate adjacent to the image in question; "hyperechoic," meaning the suspicious area shows a greater density (looks whiter on the monitor screen) than surrounding tissue; and "hypoechoic," meaning the lesion imaged is less dense (looks blacker on screen) than surrounding tissue. Sometimes, hyperechoic and hypoechoic areas can cancel each other out and a cancer could be present—even one that might be palpable—and not show up.

Dr. Cooner pioneered the use of TRUS, and his early reports on its advantages were vehemently deprecated by skeptical colleagues in academia. He persisted and was later joined by Dr. Stamey. The advent of the 7 MHz rectal probe proved Dr. Cooner's critics wrong. TRUS now is one leg of the basic tripod of diagnosis of prostate cancer, along with the PSA and the digital rectal exam. However, TRUS would be used only if DRE or PSA tests suggested cancer might be present.

Even with its advanced technology, ultrasound remains of limited use for early detection as a stand-alone method. However, a 1990 report stated that ultrasound was 75 percent accurate in identifying seminal vesicle detail, which adds to its usefulness in staging.

You Must Decide
Radiation vs. Radical

PURSUING THE SURGERY VS. RADIATION debate, as you try to decide how you wish to be treated, here is information in addition to the more generalized conclusions reported in part 1, chapter 9. I realize we are going back and forth like a tennis ball over a net, a proradiation study and then a prosurgery study and then back again. But this is the way this seemingly unresolved issue plays in the professional reports.

A 1986 report, following 682 radiated patients treated between 1973 and 1975 for ten years, shows clear benefits from radiation. Free-of-local-recurrence rates at five years were 97 percent for stage A patients, 85 percent for stage B, and 72 percent for stage C. This compares, the report said, with "the few reports of recurrence following surgery." Ten year survival rates compared generally with those of studies of surgical procedures.[1] I note that this report is somewhat dated and recurrence wasn't checked with current biopsy or PSA techniques.

A 1989 report from the University of Texas M. D. Anderson Cancer Center, Houston, discussed the "presumed superiority" of radical surgery for stages A2 and B prostate cancers. With a base of 114 patients, Drs. Gunar K. Zagars, radiotherapist, and Andrew C. von Eschenbach, urologist, reported surgical survival rates of 84 percent and 68 percent at five and ten years, respectively, comparable to the expected survival of age-matched men in the general population.

For 551 men with C cancers treated with radiation, the five-, ten-, and fifteen-year survival rates were 75 percent, 47 percent, and 27 percent. Since a lot of C patients were not considered eligible for surgery in that study's time period, no comparable surgical statistics were reported. Their conclusion was, "External beam therapy achieves overall results at least equal to those of radical surgery at five and ten years for localized prostatic carcinoma."

Not many reports have been made of fifteen-year disease-specific survival rates. Speaking to post-graduate seminars for doctors, Dr. Charles Brendler of Johns Hopkins cites one study of 70 patients with clinical stage B1 disease who underwent radical surgery between 1951 and 1963.[1] Thirteen of these could not be traced. Of the 57 remaining, the survival rate for fifteen years was 86 percent. Dr. Brendler says this indicates that only 14 percent of men with that level of disease will die of metastatic cancer in the first fifteen years following a radical prostatectomy, "if they behave like men in this study." The survival curve plateaued at ten years, indicating that men who survive for ten years following the operation are cured.

He cited a study by Dr. Malcolm Bagshaw reporting survival rates for a group of 491 patients with A2 and B cancers treated by external beam. The fifteen-year disease-specific survival was 64 percent. There was no plateau, which Dr. Brendler interpreted as meaning that men treated with radiation remained at risk of dying of prostate cancer fifteen years after treatment. A group treated with combined external beam and "seeds" had a fifteen-year survival rate of 66 percent. This shows a clear advantage of surgery over radiation, Dr. Brendler stated.

He cites a number of studies of recurrence of cancer, even though he says the various studies are difficult to compare. In them, however, recurrences were less and took longer to appear with radical prostatectomies than with radiation as initial treatment. He reported data from a Stanford study of ultrasound-guided biopsies in eighteen men who had been treated by radiation more than eighteen months previously. Biopsies were positive for sixteen of the eighteen and Brendler concludes that many if "not most patients treated with radiotherapy will have residual prostatic cancer, and such men have an increased risk of recurrence." The Stanford group performed biopsies on twenty-seven men who had radiation therapy eighteen months earlier and of twelve, ten showed PSA levels less than 10 ng/ml and had positive biopsies; all fifteen with PSA levels greater than 10 ng/ml also had positive biopsies.

A positive biopsy following radiation shows cancer is still present; it does not always mean the cancer is active (see chapter 17, in part 1, about recurrent and residual cancer). In a study at Stanford, positive biopsies after radiation for lower grade tumors (T2, T3) had no impact on survival. Of a group of nineteen patients with positive biopsies less than two years after radiation treatment, seventeen were given bone scans. Distant metastases had developed in six of them and seven had no evidence of local recurrence or distant metastases. The study also concluded that the PSA trend might be more significant than the biopsy. The study did not mention the other four patients' scans.[2]

Of course, recurring cancers will be studied and continuously assessed to see if they require a salvage procedure. Reappearance of prostate cancer following a radical prostatectomy would indicate a residual cancer, microscopic cells extended into tissues beyond the prostate and its accompanying organs that were excised in the operation.

Know More about External Beam
Survival Times by Stage

THE EFFECT OF RADIATION on cancer cells is not to incinerate them nor fry them to oblivion. The effect, when radiation works, is to damage the bad cells' capacity to reproduce themselves, to destroy them by immediate or gradual mutation so that the "children" or the "grandchildren" of the originally zapped cells become, cellularly speaking, sterile and the line dies out.

I was injected with Lupron for two months prior to my radiotherapy. My first data with the LINAC was delayed for about thirty-five days after the second shot so cells lulled into inactivity by the androgen agonist would resume whatever their nature intended. Radiation is thought to be more effective against active cancer cells. However, it will be effective, anyway; the stopping of cellular reproduction may just take longer.

There's no study comparing sets of patients on whom blockage was ceased prior to radiation and those who continued blockage right up to their meeting the LINAC. Whether the cells are dividing relatively swiftly or whether they take longer, the cells' innate sensitivity to radiation gets them eventually. Some may take six months to succumb to the radiation, some more, some less. Regression of the cancerous cells if they are slow growing could take as long as a year. The purpose of treatment is to control the cancer. Once control is established, time isn't that important. This explains also, in part, why PSA readings decline more slowly following radiation than following surgery. And, just to prove Cy Nash's "nothing's 100 percent" rule again, some cells may be immune to xrays. These could be the villains of recurrence.

You know now that radiation, despite its long and continued use, is another of those controversial subjects in prostate cancer treatment. Dr. Arthur T. Porter, professor and chairman of the Department of Radiation Oncology at Wayne State University School of Medicine, commented that of patients with organ-confined prostate cancer, stages A and B, only a minority will have their eventual outcome modified by either radiation or surgery. What he's saying is that no one has proved the treatment makes a difference in survival time. He regards both methods as "equi-potent." (See chapter 27 for more details on radiation vs. surgery.) Score one for the "no treatment" argument but not for the quality-of-life debate.

In his judgment, radiation offers fewer and milder side and after-effects. He notes that in both therapies, with advances in radiotherapy and the development of nerve-sparing surgical procedures, morbidities have changed for the better. With radiation, complications are less than 2 percent and potency retention is between 40 and 60 percent, depending on age and previous condition of potency.

In large volume, stage C, cancers he finds ten-year survivals between 30 and 40 percent. However, newer techniques may change that. In meta-static patients, radiotherapy will reduce symptoms and improve healing of damaged bone about 70 percent of the time. Improvement in implants and the use of proton radiotherapy and/or conformal external beam therapy increase the radiation dose to diseased cells. These innovations involve the technical nature of the radiation beams themselves.

The linear accelerator marked a great advancement over previous radiation technology. Dr. Malcolm A. Bagshaw and three of his colleagues from the Stanford School of Medicine summarized in *Urologic Clinics of North America,* November 1990, the rather brief history of radiation therapy.

The first try was about 1915. In 1922 the insertion of radium needles in the prostate was tried at Memorial Hospital in New York. Dr. Bagshaw said it isn't clear why radiation wasn't pursued more vigorously in those years although the Mayo clinic reported a series of treatments in 1922. Xrays prior to World War II lacked the power to deliver tumor-killing doses to internal organs without damaging skin and tissues in between.

During that time period, the basic discovery that prostate cancer was responsive to hormonal treatment diverted attention from radiation until well into the 1950s when deeply penetrating megavolt cobalt-60 and linear accelerator machines came on the scene.[1] Since few irradiated patients were subjected to autopsies, Dr. Bagshaw notes, it was difficult to prove conclusively that radiation alone had killed their cancers. He was speaking of deaths long after treatment. Some researchers maintained—and still do—that xrays rarely sterilize prostate cancers completely, yet another prostate cancer controversy.

Incidentally, certain types of cells seem to resist hormonal treatment, too.

Data is being collected on patients who require further treatment following surgery. Researchers want to see if treatment with both hormones and radiation defeats what may be a recurring cancer. In some cases, the combination works well.

Comparing the survival of patients for a given number of years, you will find survival of the radiated patients with A2 and B cancers, about the same as their nonafflicted age group, give or take a few percentage points. The numbers pertaining to those with more advanced cancers, unfortunately, reflect the deadliness of the disease.

Survival after the Ray Gun

Dr. Bagshaw's article in the *Urologic Clinics of North America* reported on Stanford's experience over several years with 1,031 carefully tracked patients treated with external beam radiation. The patients included A, B, and C staged cases. His survival charts showed the following:

STAGE A: five years, 87 percent; ten years, 77 percent; fifteen years, 45 percent. These figures are almost exactly the same expected survival times, ages averaged, for men with no disease. On his graph the stage A patients at five and ten yeas survived longer than actuarial averages for men without disease; at fifteen years, patients were only two or three percentage points below the expected survival time.

STAGE B1 AND B2: five years, 80 percent; ten years, about 62 percent; fifteen years, about 45 percent; on the charts, these ran five to ten percentage points below the "expected survival" line for comparable age groups in the general population.

STAGE B3: five years, about 75 percent; ten-years, about 55 percent; fifteen years, about 30 percent.

STAGE C1: five years, about 58 percent; ten years, about 37 percent; fifteen years, about 18 percent.

STAGE C2: five years, about 22 percent; ten years, about 17 percent; fifteen years, 17 percent.

I use "about" because the figures are graphed and so are not precise. These figures include death from all causes among the men in the study.

Interestingly, one patient with the most advanced stage, the equivalent of a D, was still living after 18 years, and the longest lived, 28.5 years after treatment, had been initially staged as a C. The follow-up period covered 22 years during which time, of course, a lot of men in the studies died of something else.

Wrote Dr. Bagshaw:

[Our studies show] that longterm survival rates indistinguishable from those expected from an age-matched peer group may be anticipated after x-irradiation in appropriately selected patients. . . . Selection factors that have been demonstrated to impact on longevity include clinical stage, Gleason grade and status of the lymph nodes.

It appears that more patients with early disease are being discovered by the combined use of ultrasound and prostate-specific antigen, and therefore, apparently an early disease category is being diagnosed without transurethral resection (TURP). These patients, and also those with nodular disease that is truly confined within the prostatic capsule, seem to be reasonable candidates for either radical resection or definitive x-irradiation. The optimum treatment for such patients depends on proper case selection, with prudent consideration of factors other than survival alone, *because survival compatible with that expected for an age-matched peer group appears likely in either case.* [Emphasis mine]

. . . The issue of choosing between surgery or irradiation in well selected cases is not as great in our opinion as is the issue of choosing patients for surgery whose disease is truly resectable [*meaning operable, with no cancer left at the margins of the removed prostate*]. In the past, preoperative understaging has been frequently associated with incomplete resection. Precise staging is not as critical before radiation therapy because generous treatment margins sufficient to include capsular penetration, periprostatic involvement, seminal vesicle invasion, or, in some cases lymph nodes, are standard. To be sure, long term survival after irradiation diminishes systematically with more advanced disease, but it does not fall to zero even in the most advanced stage.

Dr. Bagshaw also said that patients with more advanced stages, who have disease extended beyond the prostate and who seem too advanced for radical prostatectomy, still may have a 20 to 30 percent chance of fifteen-year survival. As the medical writers say repeatedly, disease progression seems to depend on the biologic aggressiveness of the individual cancer. This reference is to Gleason grades and ploidy.

Disease-free survival statistics following radiation seem to run in similar patterns no matter where the studies are done. Assorted reports from the University of Texas, the University of Pennsylvania, and the National Cancer Institute were approximately the same as the Bagshaw figures: free of recurrence for five and ten years, respectively, stage A, 84 and 77 percent; stage B, 66 and 40 percent; and stage C, 47 and 38 percent.

Please remember my repeated caution about survival statistics. As victims, we're entitled to them, and as people who want to see research improve survival, we encourage their pursuit. But a lot of victims die of other causes and long-range follow-up of patients such as the Stanford study is not the norm.

And to obtain even ten-year survival figures one has to start with patients treated in the early 1980s. Much has changed since then. Remember, too, that many patients were in their mid-seventies when their treatment began. Even a ten-year survival means they'd have to make it until their mid-eighties, not a mean feat even for a disease-free man. Also, various cancer centers measure differently; some checked recurrence only with DRE's, some with PSA, some with the more conclusive biopsy.

Drs. Barry E. Epstein and Gerald E. Hanks of the Fox Chase Cancer Center and, respectively, assistant professor and professor of radiation oncology at the University of Pennsylvania, evaluated radiotherapeutic management in *Ca—A Cancer Journal for Clinicians*.[2] They also reported "a low level of serious aftereffects of radiation therapy, 5 to 6 percent who required hospital treatment for some form of sequelae [aftereffects of treatment]."

They found preservation of potency at 73 percent in previously sexually active men and 43 percent in those considered borderline active. This is somewhat higher than other studies I've seen. They don't say who made the active vs. borderline determination: maybe the men themselves. That's a difficult call. Might be deeply influenced by the stimulation afforded by their sexual partners. I assume the before-and-after judgment by the participants in this accounting, given their average age as a group, involved no major change in the women concerned.

If your cancer is a stage B2, Epstein and Hanks state firmly that you should be treated by radiation, not surgery. If you have a stage C, they say encouragingly that long-term survival has been achieved for thousands of your brethren over the past three decades.

The percentage of prostate cancers treated with radiation in 1990 had changed little from 1984, for all stages. But the percentage of surgical treatments almost doubled for stages A, B, and D and more than doubled for stage C. There were 15,000 patients included in this report for 1984 and 23,000 for 1990. The category of treatment with the greatest decrease in use was "no treatment." But this was before the "no treatment" advocacy in the *Journal of the American Medical Association* in mid-1993. Yet we can see where some of the treatment controversies are headed in the increasing percentage of surgery in the statistics.

Materials for Hot "Seeds"

And How Well They Work

SOME OF US ON THE "GOOD" SIDE of the fight against prostate cancer get more interested than others in the technicalities and the medical details. The deeper I ventured, the more fascinated I became by the faceless, and frequently unnamed, people around the medical world studying, experimenting, and devising possible responses to the disease.

Take the materials used to make irradiated seeds for implantation. (Of course, irradiated materials are employed against cancers other than of the prostate.) Various isotopes (materials made radioactive) and assorted techniques have been used with the objective of battling the disease with as little side effect on the patient as possible. Practitioners have used lower-powered implants for permanent installation and higher-powered ones for temporary installation. Some of these have been used in combination with external beam therapy. For lower-dosage permanent treatment, the materials of choice have been iodine-125, palladium-103, ytterbium-169, iridium-192, and even gold-198.

For temporary installations, higher energies and higher dosages have been used with iridium-192 or high activity iodine-125. Drs. Nash and Toonkel in Miami have treated and are following patients on whom they used palladium-103, a white metal derivative of platinum. They use iodine seeds for well-differentiated tumors and palladium on moderately to poorly differentiated ones.

Some materials release their energy quickly, others slowly. Some cannot absorb and then release the same levels of energy as others. Dr. Arthur T. Porter of Wayne State University and chief of the Gershenson Radiation Oncology Center, Harper Hospital, Detroit, and his colleague Dr. Jeffrey D. Forman of Wayne State and the Detroit Medical Center, provided a prostate cancer conference in November 1992 with the following inventory of materials:

Iodine-125: high dose rate, rapid delivery, but difficulties in protecting the staff handling the implantation;

Palladium-103 (a platinum derivative): high energy and high initial dose rate; also used as a temporary implant; high success rate so far;

Ytterbium-169: another potential replacement for iodine-125, but problems as a permanent implant;

Iridium-192: high energy, intended as a temporary implant but patient may have to be confined to bed during treatment; good success rate with B2 and C stage cancers and also in combination use with external beam radiation.

Drs. Porter and Forman's interest in seeds grew out of concern over the failure rates of radiation therapy in terms of positive biopsies found (during the course of regular follow-up biopsies) from a year and half to twenty years following treatment. They quoted sources that 70 percent of patients with positive biopsies eventually develop metastases as compared to only 25 percent who have negative biopsies.

Effectiveness

A team of six researchers from the Departments of Urology and Radiotherapy at the University of California at Irvine and the Long Beach Memorial Medical Center, Long Beach, California, reviewed 81 patients who had biopsies between twelve and twenty-seven months after iridium implants combined with external beam radiation. Headed by Dr. Derrick Marinelli, they reported in the *Journal of Urology*, March 1992, that 82 percent with stage A, 92 percent with stage B1, 95 percent with stage B2, and 55 percent with stage C had negative biopsies and adequate local control of their cancers. In an unusual jot of humor for a medical journal they reported a previous experience, on which their current one was based, in which 241 patients over a seven-year period were treated by a "multitude of urologists" at their institution.

The combined procedure allowed them to deliver a high dose of radiation and spare normal tissue in the area. The iridium allowed precise dosage and minimum exposure to radiation to the medical staff doing the work. They used a special template for placement of the seeds. The external beam radiation was started two weeks after the interstitial therapy (implanting the seeds), although the more conventional procedure is to start with external beam and then implant the seeds. Not enough time has passed to assess their procedure in terms of survival, but they consider the short-term results, based on biopsies, as encouraging, indicating an effective method of local tumor control for patients not candidates for radical prostatectomies and especially for those with stage C disease.

Dr. John C. Blasko of the Tumor Institute Group of Seattle, Wash., had reported in 1991 on more than 450 patients in what he termed the largest experience in the world to that time using his particular technique, and the longest current follow-up in the United States. Dr. Blasko and associates used closed transperineal implantation of permanent radioisotopes (radioactive seeds) for early stage prostate cancers, and for more advanced ones, combined external beam with the implants. The technique in early cancers, using the isotopes alone, improved the accuracy of placement, resulted in minimal aftereffects, and offered patients the convenience of a single-session outpatient treatment.

The doctors used iodine-125 or palladium-103. Planning for the inserts was based on ultrasound studies of prostate volume with computer-generated seed distribution information and dosage strength. Transrectal ultrasound and special templates guided the insertion of the seeds and the operative incision was closed. CT scans were used for evaluation after implantation. Complications were minimal: 7 percent in the seeds-only patients and 8 percent in the combined seeds-external patients. Incontinence occurred in 6 percent of the seeds-only and in 4 percent of the combined treatment patients. Incontinence did not occur in patients who had not had a TURP previously. Among those who had, the complication rate was 24 percent.

With a median follow-up time of 3.5 years (two years for the palladium trials) the PSA response was better than previous reports in the medical literature. Dr. Blasko wrote that the "notable lack of rectal complications, particularly in the combined treatment group, attests to the accuracy and reliability of permanent installation by this method."

The method was not painful; only three patients experienced prolonged discomfort, and even that cleared up in time. Most patients resumed normal activities forty-eight hours after the implant. Which isotope to use depended on the Gleason grade of the tumor, with iodine employed for the lower ones and palladium the higher grades. Dr. Blasko cautioned that patients who had previously undergone transurethal prostatectomies faced a "profound" risk of incontinence. There was no incontinence among those who had no prior or postimplant surgery. Re-biopsy data appeared better than that in patients treated with external beam radiation only, but survival comparisons await the passage of more time for assessment.

This is an advancing technique as well as advancing technological therapy. The physicians using it also show an advancing enthusiasm for the results. Dr. Blasko wrote co-author Dr. Nash:

> although it is early, our experience with iodine has been encouraging, but also our experience with palladium has been very successful.

Therefore . . . we cannot offer any clear-cut advantage in general of one source over the other, other than economic, and for the fairly clear indication that high grade tumors should not be treated with iodine because the low dose rate of the long half-life source seems to be inadequate for these tumors, while palladium theoretically will be better.[1]

Dr. Blasko said the major drawback of palladium seeds is their cost. Iodine is much less expensive. Of course, neither doctor nor patient want a less effective treatment just because it is cheaper.

Dr. Brosman of Santa Monica, Calif., wrote us informally,

Our present results look quite good. The PSAs come down rapidly and the prostate also shrinks rapidly. We do biopsies yearly and at one we had positive biopsies on two-thirds of the patients. This number goes down to 50 per cent after two years. I do not have enough data to quote anything for three years.

Thus, it seems that palladium is effective in producing a clinical response but a cellular response is probably going to be the same as with any other type of radiation therapy. This would imply that in about seven more years we will start seeing a regrowth of these tumors. My impression therefore is that while this is excellent therapy it is not likely to be any better than external beam. If it turns out to be as good, it will be a big advance because of the ease of the treatment and the marked diminution in systemic side effects. . . . There is a lot to learn about this subject. . . . The ideal study would be to compare these implants to external beam but so far I have not been able to find anyone who is willing to undertake that project.[2]

Editorial comment on radiation therapy in the *Journal of Urology*, by Dr. William Shipley, Massachusetts General Hospital, Boston, notes that the Californians' approach is similar to one at Stanford except that Stanford adds interstitial hyperthermia (heat) to the implant treatment. Dr. Shipley remains skeptical of the technique's long-range success, however, until it can be assessed by thorough scientific comparisons with other approaches.

Patients eligible for implants are carefully selected. If they've had a TURP, seeds may not be used. If the prostate is too big, say more than 40 or 50 grams, seeds will not be used unless the prostate can first be shrunk with Lupron or with external beam radiation.

30

Further Hormonal Manipulation
Not Easy to Turn Off Testosterone

RECENT REPORTS of the Labrie group of Quebec signify a major change in theory if continued studies uphold them. Previously, it was thought that 20 to 40 percent of patients with advanced metastases did not respond to androgen control because their tumors contained cells that were "androgen independent."

This is why the recent Labrie reports, while influential, met some skepticism. But, the Canadians respond, the effect of complete androgen blockade as an initial form of treatment had never been tested. They maintain that prostatic cancer is more sensitive to androgens than previously believed. They believe that earlier success rates of 60 to 70 percent using DES (synthetic female hormone, estrogen) lulled researchers into not pursuing the subject, and that the serious side effects of estrogen treatments overshadowed the benefits of newer control methods. Now, they say, "The availability of more efficient drugs having no life-threatening side effects should greatly help the acceptance of complete androgen antihormonal therapy."

Dr. Labrie thus refutes former theories that the testes produce 95 percent of the body's testosterone compounds. Orchiectomy does cause a 95 percent reduction in serum testosterone concentrations, he wrote, but the concentration of dihydrotestosterone, the body's conversion of testosterone, in the body after castration or orchiectomy remains at about 40 percent of that of nondiseased men.

Drs. E. David Crawford and William L. Nabors, of the University of Colorado and Emory University respectively, reported on a major trial of total androgen ablation on patients with advanced prostate cancer, noting that men who present with metastatic tumors face a mean (half more and half less) survival of only 1.8 years.

Early attempts at total ablation involved removal of the adrenal glands by surgery. The adrenal glands also ordinarily produce small amounts of testosterone but increase output when the testicle source is removed or quelled. In the mid-fifties, adrenal testosterone was checked with cortisone. Eight out of ten patients had brief remissions with the cortisone, but the length was short, an average of eighty-two days.

A group of cancer study organizations reviewed 603 patients who had been staged as D2. A portion was placed on Lupron and flutamide and a portion on Lupron and placebos. Survival in the total ablation group was about seven months longer than in the placebo group, which the researchers classified, along with similar studies with similar results, as "not a huge advance but a step in the right direction."

It needs to be pointed out that most of the patients in these studies had not previously been treated with hormones nor received orchiectomies. Their median survival time was less than three years. In short, they were very sick when the total ablation trials began. Dr. Crawford is well recognized in the medical world for his studies in hormonal and chemical treatment of cancer. His reports confirmed a benefit in combined hormonal treatment, supporting Dr. Labrie's group, but the Crawford-Nabors report didn't show as extensive a benefit as Labrie's, if benefits can be read into the small volume of D2 reports available.

Also recent (1991) is an article by Dr. Marc B. Garnick, a clinical associate professor at the Harvard Medical School, Boston, Mass., in a brochure entitled *Controversies in the Management of Prostate Cancer* published by CoMed Publications. Dr. Garnick raised the question, is multiple agent hormonal therapy superior, and answers his query, yes, after examining the reasons for using one therapy as opposed to another.

But he says there has been little, if any, evidence that combined hormonal therapy leads to improvement in disease-free or overall survival in the previously untreated patient with metastatic disease. Again Labrie comes down with a definitive seven to fifteen months more of life with combination therapy even in the most serious D cancers and reports the best results on patients who have had no prior hormonal therapy.

Three Northwestern University Medical School doctors, James M. Kozlowski, William J. Ellis, and John T. Grayhack, deeply explored "early versus late endocrine therapy."[1] They list thirteen factors that seem to appear in aggressive tumors. Some of these you are familiar with and others are termed, by them, as esoteric, now determined largely in research institutions but, they think, fated to become standard in future real-world diagnostic routines.

In their summaries, they report that DNA diploid pattern stage D1 cancers treated with radical prostatectomies and immediate orchiectomies yielded a ten-year nonprogression rate of 100 percent. Nondiploid tumor patients relapsed with a 50 percent mortality over ten years. They strongly recommended that patient and physician participate in the treatment decision. After examining theories concerning possible risks of early androgen deprivation, they said "there is no experimental or clinical evidence that early androgen ablation is biologically deleterious," and that alternative drugs to DES have substantially decreased dangers of side effects. What's interesting to the layman here is that surgical removal of the prostate with metastasized (D stage) cancers apparently improves the effect of hormonal ablation although there is a long tradition opposing operations as an initial therapy if metastasis is found.

Dr. Garnick, however, is quite tentative in saying, conditionally, that "many patients can indeed have prolonged disease free survival and overall survival is increased when combination hormonal therapy is used." So he comes down for "cautious optimism" where total blockade is concerned and hopes more study and trials will firm up his opinion.

Dr. Labrie needs no further convincing. He called a combination therapy using a pure antiandrogen (flutamide) in association with an LHRH agonist or surgical castration the first and only treatment to prolong disease-free and overall survival in advanced prostate cancer and "the standard therapy for the disease." Moreover, he finds convincing data that the same combination facilitates radical prostatectomy by shrinking the prostate, emphasizing that early diagnosis and treatment offer the best possibility for improving prostate cancer survival.

Dr. David F. Paulson, of Duke University, comes through in his writings in the medical journals as a meticulous analyst and reporter. His essays weigh and balance every conceivable factor and are impressive in their scholarship and authority. In a November 1992 paper for *Advances in Urology*, after a searching rationale he concludes that combined hormonal therapies do provide a survival advantage over single therapies alone, appearing to add about six months to the median survival time.[2]

Dr. Paulson also examined the results of androgen deprivation on two groups of C stage patients, one of whom had a radical perineal prostatectomy along with hormonal treatment and the other radiation followed by androgen deprivation. Early or delayed hormonal treatment seemed to make no difference to the irradiated group. Dr. Paulson credited what progress those patients enjoyed to the androgen deprivation and not the radiation. He also surmised that part of the reasons patients "felt better" was that some of the hormonal drugs contained steroids.

Similarly, he questioned improvement in the radical prostatectomy group, after a Socratean dialogue with himself. Was it due to the surgery or to the androgen deprivation? His theoretical conclusion was in favor of the latter, but this brief summary does not do justice to his thorough and lucid thought processes.

He also commented that he found "flawed" the idea that preoperative androgen ablation pushes the original tumor mass back into the capsule. He concedes some advantage in the process but commented "it does not roll back these tumor cells into the primary tumor mass as one would a window shade."

Despite fairly general agreement that early is better than late, Dr. Paulson, dealing with studies of patients with reports of androgen ablation after surgery in patients with positive lymph nodes, concluded: "An even more convincing argument that early and delayed orchiectomy are equivalent in impact is afforded by the observation of early vs. delayed orchiectomy in patients with diploid vs. non-diploid tumors. [In both modes] the diploid patients had equivalent statistics while non-diploid patients do equivalently poorly if they are treated early or late."

Again, he felt that androgen deprivation and not the adjuvant surgical processes had the dominant impact on these patients.

Except that this information broadens our general knowledge of prostate cancer and might engage us in erudite conversation with our physicians, I'm not sure what the prostate cancer victim does with it. By the time he is locked into such a sophisticated course of treatment, he is a sick and very concerned individual, likely to feel desperately out of his depth in joining in a decision concerning his therapy. Yet, many of us have reason to be concerned that our treatment will not be as effective over the years as we would like and that we could confront such complex appraisals of our own situation in the future. And if we do not, it's interesting, to me anyway, to eavesdrop on knowledgeable doctors who haven't quite figured it all out, either.

Let's put one case of combined androgen ablation into human terms. The friend I mentioned earlier (chap. 4) whose doctor missed his prostate cancer until the patient himself requested a PSA, reported to me a year after starting combined treatment. Recall, he presented with a PSA of 110 ng/ml and two, possibly three, bone metastases. No pain. He told me his other doctor friends were outraged at the tardiness of the discovery. In any event, after that year his PSA is down to 0.07 ng/ml and he feels good. Maybe he'll make that fortunate 20 percent.

The Son of Cancer 1
Again, Your Decision May Rule

THIS CHAPTER IS AN INFORMATION MEMO for men who so far don't have to confront a prostate cancer treated once but now returned in one form or another. The diagnoses are complex, the various parameters that will help determine treatment the second time around can be confusing and heavy with technical details. The results of possible therapies depend on so many variables—the stage and grade of your original cancer, for example—the layman would be hard put to assemble a pro and con list for judging the choices available to him.

In part 1 we attempted to sketch in the major probabilities. In this part, we will augment that scan of treatments and consequences with additional data. Moreover, in the time it takes to produce this book important new information may be available to the urologist who keeps up with his conferences and his homework. A recurrence or a reawakening of a residual cancer requires a fine balancing of clinical histories and deeply informed judgment. We hope here to help you understand what the patient confronts and introduce therapeutic possibilities, as in part 1, chapter 16, of this book. We hope too, to show that in this fairly grim situation a substantial minority of men have done well and lived long, with a decent quality of life in their survival.

Recurrences usually are classified as "local" or "distant." Treatment methods will differ in each case, just as they differ in initial therapies involving local and distant cancers.

Surgery after Local Radiation Recurrence

In recent history, local recurrence after radiation failure has meant subjecting the patient to what's called salvage surgery or to hormonal blockade. In the past couple of years cryosurgery, the deep freeze, has been employed, with increasing frequency. See chapter 13 for the experience of Dr. Andrew von Eschenbach of the M. D. Anderson Center in Houston. Dr. von Eschenbach is using cryosurgery only for failed radiation patients. Dr. Timothy McHugh, St. Joseph Mercy Hospital, Ann Arbor, Mich., who has participated in the development of cryosurgical techniques, also uses the "ice" extensively in radiation salvage procedures.

Dr. Zincke, whose studies we referred to earlier, said that the Mayo Clinic found survival was influenced most by ploidy, that is, whether the cancer cells were tetraploid, diploid, or aneuploid.[1] His group at Mayo Clinic followed seventy-five patients who had salvage surgery due to failure of initial radiation treatment between 1967 and 1988. The patients covered an age range from fifty to eighty-one years and an assortment of initial cancer stages from B2 or less through D1. Sixteen had aneuploid tumors; the rest were diploid or tetraploid. The time between irradiation and the salvage surgery ranged from six to ninety-eight months, mean time forty-eight months. Adjuvant hormonal treatment was given to thirty-eight patients (61 percent)

PSA readings of 3 ng/ml or more were considered indicative of disease progression. Both progression of the cancer and deaths were related to ploidy. Progression occurred in 75 percent of those with aneuploid tumors, 34 percent with tetraploid, and 42 percent with diploid. Death rates were highest with aneuploid (50 percent), then tetraploid, 7 percent, and diploid, 17 percent. Hormonal treatment prior to salvage surgery proved important to diploid and tetraploid patients. In only one of eleven such patients did the cancer progress. Hormonal treatment did not seem to affect the outcome of aneuploid patients, Dr. Zinke reported.

More complications may be expected following salvage than original surgery. Dr. Zinke found 75 percent of the radical prostatectomy patients had no serious aftereffects. More frequently complications followed exenteration, which means removing all possibly affected tissue, not only the prostate, and thus involves considerably more extensive surgery and tissue removal than a radical. He also believes the number of patients who will fail after radiation will increase in the future mainly because more information is available as to the significance of postirradiation biopsies. They learn more; they do more to us, we hope for us.

Dr. Catalona espouses a more conservative view when discussing surgery following a case of failed radiation or surgery for clinical C and D cancers. In the March 1992 *Journal of Urology*, he editorialized:

This aggressive surgical approach is becoming so commonplace that soon it may be accepted as a "community standard" option that must be offered all patients.

There is no convincing evidence that these expanded indications for radical surgery for prostate cancer are justified. Why have they been so readily embraced by our profession? One reason is that there are no other potentially curative treatment options for these unfortunate patients. Another is that we have become proficient at performing these operations. . . . However, are these efforts reasonable and do we accomplish anything other than providing an element of false hope and postponing the inevitable acceptance of the reality of the situation?

He went on to recommend against radical surgery for most patients with clinical C and D disease or for those who have failed radiation. Dr. Catalona, I believe, wields as strong a pen as he does a scalpel.

Yet it's likely that most surgeons share Cy Nash's attitude. "Perhaps these procedures are desperate in a way, but if we can save a percentage of men who are in a desperate condition, even a small percentage, it's better than letting them all die."

Perhaps not as definitively, other controversies continue concerning this "enigmatic" disease. Perhaps surgery for radiation salvage and C and D cancers is a result of the desperation Dr. Catalona senses in his colleagues and their patients, perhaps not. In any event, more and more such surgeries are proceeding in this country. Maybe as the numbers mount the statistics on the troublesome outcomes will be changed for the better.

Another and possibly more likely future, if cryosurgery proves in time to truly quell the recurrent tumor longer than other options, is that freezing will replace surgery in radiation salvage therapies.

Treatment Following Recurrence after Surgery

In localized recurrence following initial surgical treatment, cryosurgery has been added to the options of radiation or hormonal blockade or combinations of the two. In distant recurrence, hormonal blockade is the prime and only choice of treatment, other than doing nothing.

Follow-up treatment through androgen denial could well start before any evidence of possible recurrence appears if your doctor finds any probability of residual cancer in your body. He may even ask you before your surgery, if his alarms are activated, whether you prefer to stop the cancer's testosterone fuel supply with orchiectomy (testicle removal) or drugs. Again, your informed decision comes into play. Do you want to have a shot once a month or your balls taken away?

Not an easy decision. Some men handle an orchiectomy as a matter of course: if they have to lose 'em, they lose 'em. Others see themselves deprived of their manhood. And some who agree to their removal, after their testicles are gone, suffer difficult psychological reactions, loss of self-esteem, and deteriorating relationships with their wives. Yet there is little difference in the physical result compared with remaining on drugs that are the equivalent of castration.

If you are young enough and may want children in the future you can store your sperm in a sperm bank just in case. This works, and it is not an unusual procedure for men who face this operation or for men who fear they may be maimed by accident or military action.

Whichever method you choose to block out testicular androgens, other parts of your body will continue to produce androgens. To stop the use of these you may be prescribed a flutamide, trade name Eulexin, which requires six pills a day and runs upwards of $300 per month. Maybe more. These treatments might follow distant radiotherapy recurrence, also.

The side effects of combined androgen ablation include hot flashes, loss of potency and sexual desire (not in everyone), diarrhea, nausea, *gynecomastia* (enlargement and tenderness of the breasts), and possible liver abnormalities.

In broad averages, the total androgen ablation therapy adds several months of survival for patients with advanced metastases but, as we continue to point out, about one person in five will live for a very long time under this treatment.[2]

Check the Stats

Statistics applicable to your particular situation may be available. There are so many variables we can't track them all here. Your doctor can obtain them more easily than you can. The sources, such as the Cancer Society and the NCI, regard every lay writer as a reporter, and I don't have to tell you that their responses to those persons are cautious, to say the least.

And not only are choices of corrective action, if any, important, the timing of their application is, too. Early radiation after an operation, if cause is seen, is more effective than delayed treatment. The same goes for androgen blockade.

A particularly cogent bit of advice came in one of the studies: "When treatment decisions involve equivalent therapies, quality of life may become the best or only differentiating endpoint. . . . Only the individual patient can judge the quality of his existence."[3]

The Great Screening Debate
Are We Finding Too Many Victims?

THIS CHAPTER DEALS WITH the continuing controversy over "screening," and highlights in digest form some of the trends in research that may be making headlines in the nineties. If pressure increases on Congress to fund broader-based screening, this will become a political issue. If some of the promising research leads to better informed treatment we and the country will benefit. We also examine briefly some of the research in progress on possible cures.

Should We Try to Find More Early Prostate Cancers?

What the country wants to know is whether mass screening of men with no outward symptoms of cancer is worth the cost and whether discovery of what might be negligible cancers will lead to costly and potentially harmful treatment.

Examine the history and current status of diagnosis and treatment and see if you want to just forget about your possible affliction.

And Cy Nash and I will continue to urge more exams for more men so more cancers can be found while they are curable.

The thirty-eight thousand men who will die this year of prostate cancer, at some point in the past had a small confined tumor subject to cure. Could they have been identified in time? Thousands of others have not died but suffer uncomfortable, expensive treatment and degradation of their lives. How much of that could have been prevented?

Dr. Peter Scardino in a talk to a Urological Society of America meeting said a study showed that with grade 1 tumors, progression of the disease occurred in about 5 percent of the cases; with grade 2, 25 percent, and grade 3, 50 percent, over seven years. As we now know, this is a short span, especially for a younger patient. "Without treatment," Dr. Scardino said, "the urologist is gambling that the patient will grow old and die of a cause other than prostate cancer."

In June 1992, the federal Centers for Disease Control reported cancer deaths increasing, especially among black men. The range of their study was from 1980 to 1988 and showed deaths up 2.5 percent among whites and 5.7 among blacks in those eight years. The increase was also on a per 100,000 basis, not only in raw numbers. White deaths rose to 17.3 per 100,000 and black deaths to 39.9 per 100,000, up about two points for each. This is close to the rate of increase medical researchers have predicted through the end of the century. However, there is a time-lag bias in their figures. The included years preceded wide use of PSA and the introduction of several new technologies.

A lot depends on how you juggle the statistics. In 1993, the Cancer Society's national data base compared 1974 and 1990 figures and found survival *improved* for each stage.

The federal report raised the question of the benefit of screening in view of the purported death rate increase. The *New York Times* questioned whether new and expensive tests were worth it, in terms of saving lives. Certainly the final answer to that question can't be tallied yet. A 1988 survival figure, since it usually takes a long time to die of this disease, hardly relates to screening in 1993. Indeed, no large-scale screening was undertaken until 1989.

In any event, the average time between detection and death, with treatment, underlines the fallacy of judging screening effectiveness over a short term. Moreover, even figures based on per-100,000 ratios must consider the increasing proportion of older men in the population and the expected rise in incidence of about 1.8 percent a year for that reason alone.

Dr. Howard Scher of the Memorial Sloan-Kettering Cancer Center in New York surveyed advances in prostate therapies during 1991.[1] He thinks the value of screening is becoming increasingly difficult to assess, as more men volunteer for exams, especially those showing no symptoms.

> The concern remains," he wrote, "that as more asymptomatic candidates are detected and treated with aggressive local modalities such as surgery or radiation therapy, the morbidity and mortality from treatment may outweigh the potential clinical impact of the disease on an individual patient. Considering radical surgery, the potential benefits must be weighed against a 1 percent mortality [in older patients], a 2.5 percent incidence of incontinence and a 25 percent rate of impotence.

Newer figures (1994) put mortality for men under seventy-five at .07 percent. Also, we'd propose that these negatives should be weighed against the chance of death within ten years.[2]

But the doctor begs off making a definitive statement about screening, citing several studies that show the procedures do not result in overdiagnosis and the majority of the cancers discovered are clinically relevant. He also reminds us that the more dangerous tumors, that is, the more un-differentiated ones (higher Gleason) yield lower PSA readings for their size than do lower Gleasons. This indicates that not all small tumors have low malignant potential. In any event, neither a PSA alone nor a DRE alone is enough to validate a diagnosis.

We dealt with the "no treatment" philosophy earlier in some detail but the question remains active and, indeed, the "watch and wait" viewpoint may be gaining ground. Uncertainties persist about aggressive treatments that all too often generate their own problems, but when measured by quality of life and survival time, may truly benefit patients under seventy. With men seventy-five or older no benefits are perceived, although most urologists would not perform surgery on men of that age. One of the pur-poses of this book is to help you participate in decisions about your own life; this debate deserves your full attention. And you will be asked your preference: treat or not treat.

Dr. Willet F. Whitmore Jr., whom we have quoted previously, asked for patient participation in an editorial on the subject in the *Journal of the American Medical Association* thusly: "Although any benefits of aggressive treatment over watchful waiting in terms of quality-adjusted life expect-ancy are often small in absolute terms, whether they should be considered negligible may be a decision best left to the individual patient."[3]

One of the points of contention in this critical debate concerns what level of PSA should trigger more exploratory—and expensive—testing. At PSA's under 4.0 ng/ml, for example, more biopsies and sonograms would be required to find each cancer than tests at levels greater than 4.0. In Canada, Dr. Labrie and associates screened 1,002 men selected at ran-dom from voting lists. Their "threshold" of PSA was 3.0 ng/ml. With higher readings they do further tests, DRE's and TRUS. They found can-cer in fifty-seven men, or 5.7 percent of those screened. Learning that crit-ical PSA levels can be related to age should further clarify screening tests.

Their approach, they wrote, "set the cost of diagnosis of one prostate cancer at $1500, while $30,000 is the estimated cost for diagnosis of one breast cancer by mammography." They don't suggest broad PSA screen-ing as perfect but as an effective way to find a lot of early cancers and per-haps cure them.[4]

Dr. Nash agrees that this is one way to cover a large number of poten-tial prostate cancer victims but fears Dr. Labrie will miss a number of cancers unless ultrasound and DRE's are included in the screening. Somewhere between 17 and 30 percent of cancers will not register an elevated PSA. Nevertheless, Dr. Labrie's reputation as an innovator brings quite respectful attention to his proposition.

Dr. William J. Catalona, whose Washington University Medical Center is three years into a five-year screening program that will involve 18,000 men, agrees in part with Dr. Labrie on PSA as an effective screening tool. But Dr. Catalona places the critical threshold at 4.0 rather than 3.0.

In a telephone interview, he told me that 90 percent of the men screened will have PSA's less than 4.0 and if the critical testing level used is 3.0, double the number of biopsies will be required. He estimates cancer will be present in only 6 percent of men with PSA levels between 4.0 and 3.0. Less than one in ten men in that range tested will have cancer, making the discovery of each cancer inordinately costly. "I agree," he said, "that PSA is a useful first test. But remember that the DRE and ultrasound combined are better than the PSA alone."

Dr. Gleason wrote that survival after diagnosis depends on three things: the histologic grade (the cells), clinical stage (A, B, etc.), and the age of the patient. For example, a grade $2 + 3$ (5) in a seventy-five-year-old man won't change his mortality significantly, but the same grade in a forty-five-year-old man halves his longevity. A $3 + 4$ (7) grade Dr. Gleason calls ominous at any age.

Then, could a doctor be comfortable with watching and waiting if his patient shows an A1 cancer which by definition is nonpalpable, confined to the prostate, with a low Gleason grade? That's going to depend on your doctor's philosophy and the extent of tumor revealed by a biopsy plus your life expectancy. It's generally agreed that a tumor that decides to grow will double every three to four years, although one researcher says every three to four *months*, which is unusually fast according to a consensus of doctors interviewed.

So, if your nodule is 1.5 cc now, in four years it could be 3.0. In eight years, 6.0 cc. By that time, the likelihood is that the cancer will escape the prostate capsule and invade lymph nodes and other organs. Would you like to go for twelve years? Well, you wouldn't let it go that long. The signs of progression would be so evident the "waiting and watching" would have been ended long ago. However, you would have a cancer by that time difficult to treat and perhaps impossible to cure. You would have reached a level at which survival may have been shortened.

"Tell me which ones to watch," Dr. Nash says. "I can't tell. I don't want to watch you until you are in pain and have metastases in your bones. I'd rather treat you when I have a good chance of curing you."

I have reported the screening argument at length because Cy Nash and I want to reply to it with a sentence: "What if the cancer detected is in *me?*"

For one thing, no one is advocating a sweeping and continuing screen of every man over fifty in the entire world, even in the United States. For another, given the ambition for such a mass screening, not every male could be checked in one year or even ten. Every urologist's finger in America would be worn down to the nub. No hospital parking lot could handle the jam. The idea is to screen high-risk portions of the population, men who are concerned about themselves, men with family histories of prostate cancer or other prostate problems. I have read no proposal for sending out examination trailers to park on street corners and dragoon passersby in for blood tests or TRUS exams. Some day there might be a quick and easy test. Not now.

But screening by hospitals and existing centers could be expanded for modest cost. Screening goes on all over the country now. A typical program is at Mr. Sinai Hospital on Miami Beach although many other hospitals have similar projects, especially during National Prostate Cancer Awareness week. Mt. Sinai advertises a phone number in the local supplement to the *Miami Herald.* The hospital public relations staff handles the calls and books appointments. The doctors in the urology department donate their time, maybe two to four hours a day. The hospital provides orange juice and coffee for the examinees and pays for the PSA test.

The hospital and the Comprehensive Cancer Center share costs and one of the labs gives a basic cost rate for the PSA tests, around $14 compared to a regular fee of about $50. Cy says, "The people get their blood drawn, someone takes a brief history and they go into a room and get a quick rectal exam. We don't get into a lot of things; just the rectal, the PSA, and a little bit of 'How you doing?' It takes about a couple of weeks to get all the test results back. I go over them, 350 of them last time, with help from the staff. The ones that have a suspicious rectal or a PSA over 4.0 whether the rectal was suspicious or not, get a letter from us urging them to have a further workup.

"We're especially interested in younger people. That's where the real trouble is prevented. That's where we are going to improve their chances. The argument that screening will create a lot of unnecessary treatment or morbidity I can't agree with. If you are one of the guys we pick up, it could save your life. So, what does 'cost effective' mean? The doctors donated their time, the hospital and the Center didn't charge anything, the lab was cheap. No one has to pay for every step of a screening program.

"Really, we do screening all the time. If some one comes to the office with any kind of symptom, the incidence of finding prostate cancer will be higher than in a general screening. So the yield will be higher. But by that time, the patient will also be in much greater danger. If you look at the question in purely economic terms, look at what you save by catching it early, including possibly preventing death."

Some modest support from foundations or the government to increase the screening that can be performed in ways similar to the national procedure—and several Miami hospitals do this—could save lives and, by minimizing treatment, dollars as well. During National Prostate Cancer Awareness Week, cancer centers and hospitals across the country run screening programs. This is not a new idea, but it needs further expansion.

Intensified screening in low income communities could save considerable pressure on already beleaguered families and their men. As a veteran of assorted civic activities I can easily imagine local organizations set up around the country as offshoots of a national prostate cancer society, or even as branches of local American Cancer Society units. These could sponsor broader community screening programs through cooperation with urology societies and local hospitals without waiting for a special "week" each year. It should not be difficult to raise funds locally for screening if everyone concerned pitched in. We're raising money for everything else.

33

A Look at the Future
So, What Else Is New?

WHEN PROGRESS AGAINST PROSTATE CANCER seems bleak and it looks as though there's nowhere else to go, along comes a group that finds and develops PSA testing or improves the use of sonograms or adds to the effectiveness of xrays. In the past ten years innovators in cellular biology and genetics or avid students of anatomy and surgical techniques have changed the course of prostate cancer discovery and treatment.

For example: increased understanding of PSA, acceptance of early androgen ablation, the nerve-sparing surgical technique, cryosurgery, new seed implants, major advances in understanding the whole process of how cancers spread themselves in the body, laparoscopy in lymph node dissection and on and on. To say that none of these have or will decrease the prostate cancer death rate, as did a recent NCI report, is too pessimistic. There are still critically important questions unanswered but to surrender to an enigmatic biological imperative posed against us by cancer is unthinkable.

Take a look at obscure—at least to the public at large—searches going on now:

PIN as an Early Warning

It's a given that as the population ages there'll be more prostate cancers. It is also a given that the aggressiveness of an early prostate cancer is difficult to detect. So diagnosticians show sharp interest in two lesions of the prostate that are called "precancerous," and suggest cancer is either in the offing or somewhere other than the biopsy location.

These are "prostatic intraepithelial neoplasia" (new growths) referred to as PIN and "atypical adenomatous hyperplasia," referred to as AAH. PIN as a name is recognized by international conferences and is standard. There are stages of PIN, as there are of prostate cancer. Primarily PIN shows up as groups of crowded, heaped up and irregularly spaced cells. There're PIN I and PIN II, for low grade and high grade. High grade means cancer is nearby, perhaps adjacent to the PIN II site. It may show up in biopsies, TURP tissues, or removed prostates, either in company with cancer or as a precursor to cancer. AAH isn't quite so definitively associated with cancer, but most researchers consider it a marker for later development of cancer.

PIN is an important signal to the pathologists analyzing tissues because it is a sure warning sign. Currently PIN is not being treated directly: it is an alerting signal. Also, through tracking PIN, researchers hope to learn more about how cancer develops. No one's going to stick needles in you to find PIN specifically; such findings are coincidental to biopsies and TURPs, in most cases.

How Smart Is a Cancer Cell?

Donald S. Coffey, Ph.D., of Johns Hopkins points out that normally the body's cells are in balance: some die, new ones are born. A cancer tumor is a result of imbalance in the birth rate and death rate. Johns Hopkins researchers are trying to figure out why some cells die and some grow. If cell death could be regulated, a balance might be restored.

Johns Hopkins also is seeking to identify the molecular mechanisms that cause cancer cells to move. If this mobility could be blocked somehow metastases could be stopped before they start.

Dr. Lance Liotta, M.D., Ph.D., chief of the pathology lab at the National Cancer Institute and colleagues, concentrating primarily on breast cancer, are also working on how tumor cells spread through the body undetected and invade distant organs.[1] They reported that less than one in 10,000 tumor cells that leave the primary tumor survive to start new tumor colonies. These travel in lymph and blood fluids and anchor themselves in new sites. They then create their own blood supply. They manage to pierce the protective level of cells that line blood and lymph vessels and penetrate what are called cellular "basement membranes" in healthy cells. The invading cells must "bore a tunnel, grip the sides of the tunnel and propel themselves forward" to anchor in a new position. These are the steps in metastasis, or tumor extension in the body.

Dr. Liotta's group found that high metastatic tendencies were associated with the presence of a class of enzymes that manage to separate protective protein layers and permit tumor cell invasion of new sites. They call these enzymes "metalloproteinases." So, at each step in the metastatic process there may be ways to block the cancer cell in its mission. Stop the cleavage of protective cells; stop the travel of bad cells; stop the action of the metalloproteinases. The researchers are excited about checking the spread of tumors by interrupting their action at any of these steps.

There may be a substance present, also, that overwhelms the bad cells.

It is called TIMP-2. If there is enough of it present it can halt the cell inva-sion process, or it can block the formation of new blood vessels that nourish the new cancer cell colony. (One of the ways tumors kill people is by demanding so much nourishment the body cannot sustain both the tu-mors and itself and in effect dies of starvation.)

As this work becomes more public, you'll probably hear of the "nm23 gene." High levels of "nm23," seem to discourage metastasis. The original work on nm (standing for nonmetastatic) 23 was in connection with breast cancer, but it has been observed in studying other forms of cancer, as well.

Also, Dr. Liotta's group has started clinical trials with a class of syn-thetic compounds that may stop the growth of human tumors, including prostate tumors.

I find the pursuit of knowledge about genetics and cancer a fascinating subject even if the technicalities and the discussions of altered chromo-somes and so-called p53 tumor genes, which may have the ability some-times to suppress cancer, grow too complex for someone not thoroughly trained in that field.

Indeed, I wonder if the final answer to cancers may not arise from bio-genetic studies that lead to manipulating the body's own healthy cells to prevent or conquer tumors. I asked one urologist (not Nash) if he thought genetics might provide the ultimate answer to prostate cancer before any of the other lines of research did so. "No," he said, flatly. I'm not that sure.

Perhaps cells have much more to tell us. One of the great puzzles in prostate cancer has to do with determining which cells have the most dan-gerous metastatic potential. If urologists could tell that, probably a sizeable portion of early cancers could, indeed, remain untreated with no fear of their spreading. Researchers are studying the shape of cancer cells, espe-cially their "roundness," to discover whether the shape of the cell and its nucleus can foretell its virulence.

Urine PSA Tests May Be Easier and More Accurate than Blood Serum Tests

With the remarkable information available from testing for specific prostatic antigen (PSA) in blood serum, not a cheap process, maybe there's a noninvasive way to perform the test. Dr. Ralph W. de Vere White and associates from the University of California, Davis, announced that PSA levels can be as accurately obtained from urine as from blood serum. They published their findings in the March 1992 *Journal of Urology.*

They found in some critical cases, following radical prostatectomies for stages A to C cancers, for example, that of forty-three patients 77 per-cent had elevated urinary PSA's while only 33 percent had elevated serum levels. What this meant to them is that close to 80 percent of the patients had tumor-bearing prostate tissues remaining locally after the operation, and the standard tests didn't identify them.

The team said it could find only one prior reference to urinary PSA levels in the literature. Their study set out to test their hypothesis that urinary PSA's could be valuable. Some possibly interesting detective story plot twists appeared in their studies, too. For instance, testing urine samples from female volunteers, they found that those who had had sexual intercourse within twenty-four hours of urine collection showed elevated levels of PSA. The other female volunteers showed 0.0 to 0.4 ng/ml and had not had intercourse within twenty-four hours. They were not asked how long it had been since they had. Possibly the lower PSA's represented a longer time since intercourse. An early study referred to had shown that in rape victims—more detective work—PSA can be detected up to forty-eight hours in urine samples. Remember, women cannot produce PSA by themselves.

PSA was equally as accurate in frozen urine samples, an important finding in terms of storing samples for future analysis. Since PSA levels are higher in the first urine voided after ejaculation, Dr. White's team was not surprised to note that such testing was first investigated in connection with rape. They found, too, that after the first voiding following ejaculation, the PSA returned to a base line.

Most men's urinary PSA's matched probable blood serum PSA's under comparable circumstances, except following surgery. The finding that following radical prostatectomies urine PSA elevations were more than twice as common as elevated blood serum PSA's, suggested to Dr. White's team that residual cancer may be present in more patients than has been previously suspected. More study will be required before the team is ready to say that postoperative clinical treatment will be required for men whose urine PSA is up but whose blood serum PSA is not.

If urinary analysis of PSA proves consistently accurate it should reduce the cost of testing because a technician would not be required to draw blood and specimen handling would be cheaper.

However, if you were looking for a new scientific twist in your next detective novel now you have a heretofore unused gimmick.

Biological Warfare: Helping the Genes Do Their Work

The field of biotechnology may one day come up with the most effective answer to cancer, including that of the prostate, but no one's sure when. The molecular biologists, immunologists, and geneticists already know that there are genes that can suppress cancer, genes that encourage cancer growth, and genes that bolster the body's own immune system to fight bad cells when they show up.

We have tumor-suppressor genes that can make tumor-causing genes inactive. We also have oncogenes that can cause mutations of other genes.

Researchers in diabetes, for example, think that the body's immune system actually destroys the "beta cells" in the pancreas that produce insulin. They hope to analyze by genetic screening those genes that control or regulate the immune system and so identify people at the greatest risk of developing insulin-dependent diabetes. Maybe then, they can interfere with the process and prevent diabetes before it develops.

A genetic scientist, speaking to a conference in Houston in 1993, summed it up: "Our aim will be to identify the genetic abnormality that predisposes patients to prostate cancer, screen for that abnormality, and then correct it by directly replacing genes in the prostate. Through this kind of therapy, we feel the problem of prostate cancer will be defeated."

Looking for the Cancer-killing Chemical

Basically, the researchers are looking for something to use on advanced cancer patients when hormonal treatment fails. They call this "hormone-refractory" disease. The drug Ketoconazole, for example, reduced PSA levels in a high proportion of patients and eased their cancers but did not prolong survival.

Another drug, Suramin, has evoked some response in disease repression, but is quite toxic and the experts are not sure yet how to administer it, intermittently or with prolonged exposure. In the lab it does show significant ability to kill cancer cells. One testing group that combined Suramin with hormonal treatment reported significant drops in PSA readings and better tolerance of the Suramin. Suramin limits the growth of malignant cells and has produced some limited success in hormone-refractory patients. Some gains in reducing toxicity have been reported. In the *Yearbook of Urology 1993* co-editor Dr. J. Y. Gillenwater termed it "one of the best chemotherapeutic agents we have to use against hormone resistant cancer of the prostate." If its toxic impact can be controlled, Suramin would be good news, because no really effective chemical that is worse for the cancer than for the patient has been identified.

Finasteride (Proscar) is building a record in treating BPH (enlarged prostate), but it must be taken for a long time to achieve results. It has not been effective against prostate cancer in single therapy modes but may be in combination with some hormonal treatments. It interferes with the body's use of testosterone. Its advantage is that it produces minimal side effects. A major national test involving eighteen thousand men for seven years is underway now to see if it can prevent cancer.

Chemical researchers are looking for two things: one is a compound useful when tumors resist or seem to be immune to hormonal treatment; the other is a direct cancer cell killer (cytotoxic) that doesn't rough up the patient. Chemicals have been successful sometimes against other cancers but nothing specific to prostate cancer has worked so well that anyone is touting it. Hundreds have been tried but only two seem to have worked at least 20 percent of the times used. These were Vinblastine and EmCyt, tested experimentally at Memorial Sloan-Kettering after patients relapsed following total androgen ablation and/or Suramin.

The Future

With growing political awareness of prostate cancer, especially in the Senate where more aging legislators are vulnerable to the disease, more research money should be forthcoming. As the third leading cancer killer in the United States, just behind breast and lung cancer, prostate cancer falls well down the list in financial support.

But prostate cancer victims are becoming better organized, and in the early nineties funds purposed specifically to raise money for prostate cancer research emerged. The accumulation of statistics in quantity to help analyze the variety of therapies and combinations of therapies discrete for the various stages has lagged, as well as funding. As the newer treatment modes build years of experience they must be tracked in statistical detail in order to be reasonably judged.

Some of the gurus see the fairly new procedure of checking PSA density providing more guidance to surgeons and radiotherapists alike. Dr. Carl A. Olsson, Columbia University and chair of the department of urology at Columbia Presbyterian Medical Center, New York, following a study of one hundred prostatectomies, said if the PSAD was 0.35 or less, surgical cures were about 90 percent; near 0.6, cures fell to 33 percent. At the 0.35 level radiation successes were the norm, while at 0.6 failures were 100 percent.

Dr. Olsson expects more radical prostatectomies in the future, replacing TURPs as surgeons' most common procedure.

During a recent visit to Miami, Dr. Murphy told us he and his associates are trying to isolate two types of PSA, one for malignant and one for benign tissue, in order to separate BPH and cancer analysis.

Literally hundreds of tests and research projects are in progress. Most of them are specific and detailed, if narrowly financed. Better communications among researchers and practitioners hope to bring worldwide experiences into some sort of coherence.

The last ten years have seen more progress in prostate cancer study and treatment than in the entire history of the disease. The next ten will be even more impressive.

A Little Catching-Up Time

IT'S TAKEN FAR TOO LONG to prepare this book. In that time, with my initial presentation in late 1989 and radiation treatment in early 1990, the damn thing recurred. I am now in the statistics as a "failed radiation" patient. And I have yet to feel any pain or any other awareness of the cancer except for tests that proved positive.

My PSA scores rose from 0.7 in late 1990 to 3.0 ng/ml in late 1992. Two subsequent six-month PSA's were level and in December 1993 the test rose to more than 5.0. Cy Nash examined me, felt the returning hardness of the tumor and on biopsies found the proof of recurrence, with a Gleason grade up from my original 7 in 1989 to 8.

For the first time since all this started I felt a deep wave of concern. Until the recurrence my mental attitude had been calm. I simply resolved to go the course of treatment, lost my self in studying and writing about prostate cancer, wondering as deadlines neared whether I had bitten off more than I could chew. But I held to my schedules for the future: leisurely writing the book of newspaper reminiscences I've been promising for years, minor travel, summers in the hills, easy social times with friends, tending my grapes and maybe being a little more scientific in putting up some wine in the fall, maybe getting around to promoting this book when we finally finished it. I was not frightened. I've accommodated to the ultimate.

I suppose I simply started taking this cancer more seriously. It was aggressive, no doubt about that. Now, I began to see it as more than an inconvenience, rather as a permanent and perhaps implacable enemy that would no longer consent to being a side issue in my life but a central fact that would set my agenda and put new constraints on my freedom. It had to be quelled.

So, what to do?

Wait? Two advisors suggested that. What would I be waiting for with such an active tumor? For the PSA to go to 10? Fresh tests, CT scans, and bone scans showed no metastases. According to these, the tumor was still locally contained, at least not extended. I could wait. But I thought I knew too much. I didn't want any more suspense than necessary in my life.

Suppose it exploded between routine PSA tests. I'd have limited options, probably total androgen ablation. At that point, I could start immediately on an LHRH agonist and an antiandrogen. Or, I could have an orchiectomy and antiandrogens, which would have been my choice, and may have to be in the future. Such therapies for far more advanced cancers have been successful for various lengths of time, but I did not want to risk the possible side effects of any of these until forced to do so. What were my other options?

A salvage radical prostatectomy? While there've been some good results, in most follow-up reports 25 percent of such operations produced a range of troublesome aftereffects. One doctor, Paulson of Duke, has reported far better success than that. Another, Catalona of Washington University, classified salvage radical prostatectomies among the therapies he considers excessively risky. Cy Nash, my immediate guru and expert, did not favor that course and, as self-anointed self-diagnostician, I didn't like it, either.

A second round of radiation? Just not done. Implanted seeds? Possible, but with prior radiation plus a TURP in my history an invitation to trouble, too much chance of permanent incontinence. Besides, my confidence in radiation therapy understandably had diminished.

Think about the ice, Cy suggested. Mt. Sinai hospital recently had installed the CMS cryosurgery five-probe gear. I had added a chapter about it to this book. Recent studies were favorable. What the "deep-freeze" lacked was that five years or more of history for at least preliminary scientific verification of the process that medicine wants before it dives into wholesale utilization of a new technology.

Andrew von Eschenbach, M.D., of the M. D. Anderson Cancer Center in Houston revealed to us his team's record of almost one hundred cryoablations of radiation-failed patients. He and his colleagues showed increasing good results. (See chap. 13.) My own doctor Cy Nash had taken a short course in cryosurgery in Pittsburgh where the new five-probe procedure was developed. One of his instructors there was Timothy McHugh, M.D., of St. Joseph Mercy Hospital in Ann Arbor, Mich. Cy knew that McHugh was planning a trip to Florida.

At this time the Mt. Sinai crew with its machine barely out of the wrappings was early in its cryosurgical experience, especially with previously radiated patients. Besides, our personal relationships during the preparation of this book had become too close. And I wanted a surgeon who had accrued as much experience with the process as I could find. By coincidence, Dr. McHugh had another patient in south Florida awaiting his ministrations. Dr. McHugh agreed to "do" me.

He appeared in my hospital room the evening before the procedure. I had been "prepped," meaning an attendant had shaved me vigorously, front and rear, throughout the pubic area, from belly-button to tailbone, and the anesthesiologist had interviewed me. Dr. McHugh, who appeared to be in his mid-forties, was pleasant and friendly after his long trip and told me not to worry about a thing. All would go well.

I came out of anesthesia while they were dumping me from the trundle cart onto my hospital bed. Anne greeted me with love and cheers, obviously glad I had come around to consciousness again, with the cancer, we hoped, frozen and thawed into oblivion. Cy had assisted Dr. McHugh. He showed up soon and said the procedure went very well.

There was a little tube sticking out of my lower abdomen. It had a "T" valve connected to another tube, which extended into a plastic bag strapped to my left thigh. I was voiding urine into the bag. Within the hour, I walked to the bathroom and opened a stopper valve on the bag and drained it into the toilet. It began to fill again. Cy showed me that by turning the "T" valve, urine would be diverted from the plastic bag and would be voided through my own, exclusively personal equipment. He said I could go home if I wanted, with the bag.

"Oh, no," Anne said. "I'm not ready for that." Anne was recovering from her own medical ordeal, a lumpectomy. When it rains, it pours, in our family. Nursing a guy and his urine bag through the night ranked low on her agenda. She had her own problems to take care of. So I stayed another night in the hospital, a total of three nights. Amazing.

The next morning, we turned the valve and I voided on my own, a weak stream bringing a slight burning and carrying a pinkish tinge. Cy relieved me of the bag but left the tube protruding, just in case. Still no real pain. I could feel sutures (which would in time dissolve away) sticking out of my crotch.

"You can shower, eat whatever you like. Try to urinate every couple of hours and see how your control goes. Go do whatever you feel like doing," Cy instructed me, adding some antibiotic (Cipro) to my diet to override any chance infection.

"They" don't let any patient walk out of a hospital. I rode a wheelchair to the front door, Anne drove up in her car. I got into the car gingerly, still expecting something to hurt but except for the crotch punctures where the five probes had been inserted into my prostate, nothing did. Some mild analgesic, Darvocet or something, managed that pain efficiently.

The next morning at his office Cy removed the T-valve and tube. He put a bandage slightly larger than a Band-Aid over the little hole where the tube had been and that, to quote Winnie the Pooh, was that.

He reviewed the operation for me. The five tubes went in with only small surgical cuts to ease their passage through my crotch skin. The monitor showing ultrasound pictures displayed the location of the probes and the "iceballs" they created. My urethra was warmed with a flow of body-temperature water. Dr. McHugh introduced liquid nitrogen into the tubes and the resulting freezing appeared to cover the entire prostate. He withdrew the tubes a few centimeters, shifting their position slightly, and repeated the freezing and thawing. Cy showed me a series of pictures of the ultrasound monitor, recorded throughout the process. Looked OK to me. The probes seemed well distributed as far as I could tell.

For a few days I walked as though I had been horseback riding the Chisholm Trail. My scrotal wall swelled to triple size, not painfully, and turned blue-black from blood draining into it. Ten days after the operation it had returned to normal and I restarted my simple, and short, morning exercises. The sutures were gone. When the urge struck, I could not delay dashing to the bathroom, but I could feel normal control returning. I felt I really should go to the range and hit a bucket of golf balls. Tomorrow, I decided.

The object of all this, of course, was to kill the tumor for good. I would have PSA tests once a month for three months and, at the third, would be biopsied again. Regular tests would continue at intervals.

Nothing about this is fun. Hospitals are not recreational. But compared to other procedures, with the possible exception of radioactive implants, cryosurgery proved to be relatively painless and not too disruptive of one's regular activities. The big question is, did it eliminate the tumor? Radiation stultified the bad cells for four years, in my case. We'll see how long the "ice" keeps them at bay. After all, this is one process that can be repeated if it doesn't work the first time, not that I'm looking forward to it.

I will have periodic tests for a while, another biopsy in about three months. I still don't know if the "ice" will work as advertised, nor for how long it will be effective. My concerns did ease. I put on my "What? Me worry?" face. Still feeling a little fragile, eleven days after the procedure I went to the range and swung my golf club nice and easy, smooth as ice. I hit the ball a ton. I'd been looking for that swing for a long time.

Notes

Chapter 2

1. If even a small percentage, say a third, of TURP's could be avoided by use of drugs or laser surgery, the savings in national health costs could be enormous. A TURP costs from $8,000 to $10,000 depending on the hospital. Eliminating 100,000 a year would save approximately $800 million to $1 billion annually, not adding back in the cost of the alternative procedures, which are far less costly.

2. John Kabalin, M.D., an editorial, *Journal of Urology* 150 (Nov. 1993):1749–50.

3. Monroe Greenberger, M.D., and Mary Ellen Siegel, M.S.W., *What Every Man Should Know about His Prostate* (New York: Waler and Co., 1983; rev. ed., 1988).

4. To underscore the range of opinions in this field, I am further informed that this "fluid theory" is "urologic folklore" and has no basis in scientific fact. You can see why I found this study intriguing. Is your doctor a "folklorist" or does he/she agree with the several references to this matter I have read? Or, you may look to your own, perhaps youthful, experiences.

5. One of my friendly reader-helpers said that when she heard this joke the doctor was eighty-five.

Chapter 3

1. See chapter 26, in part 2, for further information on ultrasound (U/S). It is an important scientific tool, but I do not want to interrupt our narrative here with notes long enough to do U/S justice. PSA will be explained further, also.

2. See chapter 7 for information gained from "flow cytometry" and other analyses by microscope of your cancer cells. Dr. Gleason developed this measurement scale. It will be an important part of your diagnosis. Both your "grade" and "stage" are critical determinants of your possible treatment, so we go into extensive detail about them later on.

Chapter 4

1. PCa is shorthand for prostate cancer, which in doctors' slang is sometimes also referred to as "CA of the prostate."

2. We'll return to the treatment and follow-up in this example later on. There was an amazing coincidence in this instance. After all these years, we learned my former shipmate lives only a block from the home of my younger son near Princeton, N.J.

Chapter 5

1. Although we had no MRI reading, since my tests I've learned that the magnetic resonance pictures of prostate cancer have improved considerably because of the development of new "endorectal" (meaning inside the rectum) coils to be used in the process. These bring the coils in closer proximity to the prostate and result in better definition of the pixels, the tiny dots on a screen that add up to pictures. In MRI, unlike the CT, the pixels can be manipulated by computer for various views of what it sees. MRI may be able to confirm whether cancer has invaded the seminal vesicles. It might be important in revealing the size of lymph nodes and examining the area near the capsule. So far, these expectations haven't been fully realized.

2. Following surgical removal of the prostate, cancer recurrence, if any, usually arises from undetectable microscopic cells remaining in the "margins" of the operation, those tissues adjacent to the former location of the prostate. One of the reasons for radiation is that the rays can cover the entire region and may kill marginal cells.

Chapter 6

1. In a way, the first time you visit your urologist you are being screened, but the term usually describes a process for testing large numbers of the male population. The extent of screening advocated by doctors who think there ought to be a lot of it across the cancer-susceptible age group is a controversial subject.

2. More technical information is in part 2.

3. A centimeter is 0.4 inches, four-tenths of an inch, that is.

4. Prostatic acid phosphatase, in longer use than the PSA, also measures prostate disturbances but is not as accurate and reacts to a wider range of problems than the PSA. It is usually referred to as PAP. It is now used primarily as an indicator of bone or soft tissue spread (metastasis) and is reliable to about 70 percent. A rising PAP generally means a stage D cancer and treatment for a localized cancer is not used.

Chapter 7

1. J. Y. Gillenwater, M.D., *Yearbook of Urology, 1993*, p. 178.

2. I'm trying to focus on direct patient diagnostic matters here, so please refer to chapter 26 in part 2 for a fuller discussion of PSA and its general importance in cancer analysis and treatment. What to do about PSA's in the 4 to 10 ng/ml range is a major topic among physicians.

3. Interview with Dr. Joseph E. Oesterling, Mayo Clinic, *Urology Times*, Sept. 1993, pp. 13–22. New interpretations of PSA levels, including the relationship of PSA and age, may also help doctors decide which patients may be treated with "watchful waiting" and which require immediate treatment. We tackle this decision controversy in the next chapter.

4. Jerome P. Richie, M.D., et al., "Effect of Patient Age on Early Detection of Prostate Cancer with Serum Prostate-Specific Antigen and Digital Rectal Examination," *Urology* 42, no. 4 (Oct. 1993): 365–374.

5. Joseph E. Oesterling, op. cit.

6. The patterns identified in the Gleason scale start with 1, a collection of cells that look alike, are clearly outlined, regular in shape and differentiated from one another. At level 5, the cells are irregular in shape and size and are not differentiated from

each other. If you could look through the microscope you'd have no trouble distinguishing between a 1 and a 5. It is apparent that a grade 2 + 3 (Gleason 5) tumor in a seventy-five year-old man would not increase his mortality risk drastically. But the same tumor in a forty-five year-old man halves his expected survival time. Dr. Gleason wrote that actuarial data can be combined with "cancer specific death rates for a certain tumor grade to produce a theoretical survival curve for a group of such patients."

7. Remember, if you are easily nauseated you may ask for the costlier nonionic medium.

8. A current commentary in the *Journal of Urology* states that though it is too early to define the absolute reliability of new MRI coils they offer "great promise" and show an accuracy of 82 percent in differentiating between stages B and C cancer, a remarkable improvement over the digital exam. A half a cubic centimeter would be about the size of a small pea.

9. For more detailed information on testing and grading, see part 2. Even deeper reading and a full array of charts and statistics on these items can be obtained from the National Cancer Institute, the *Journal of Urology*, or various monographs, including, on PSA particularly, the *1989 Monographs in Urology*, volume 10, no. 4, published for Merck and Co., West Point, Pa., by Medical Directions Publishing Co., Inc., PO Box 3000, Princeton N.J. 08534, contents copyrighted by Thomas Stamey, M.D., of Stanford.

Chapter 8

1. Craig Fleming, M.D., John H. Wasson, M.D., Peter C. Albertson, M.D., Michael J. Barry, M.D., John W. Wennberg, M.D., M.P.H., for the Prostate Patients Outcomes Research Team, "A Decision Analysis of Alternative Treatment Strategies for Clinically Localized Prostate Cancer," *JAMA*, vol. 269, no. 20 (May 26, 1993), pp. 2650–2658; Grace L. Lu-Yao, Ph.D., M.P.H., Dale McLerran, M.S., John Wasson, M.D., and John E. Wennberg, M.D., M.P.H., "An Assessment of Radical Prostatectomy: Time Trends, Geographic Variation, and Outcomes," ibid., pp. 2633–2636; and Willet F. Whitmore Jr., M.D., "Management of Clinically Localized Prostatic Cancer" (editorial), ibid., pp. 2676–2677.

2. "Therapeutic Options in the Management of Incidental Carcinoma of the Prostate," *International Journal of Radiation: Oncology, Biology, Physics*, vol. 20 (1991), pp. 153–167.

3. Jan Adolfsson, M.D., Gunnar Steineck, M.D., and Willet F. Whitmore, Jr., M.D. "Recent Results of Management of Palpable Clinically Localized Prostate Cancer," *Cancer*, vol. 72, no. 2 (July 15, 1993).

Chapter 9

1. Deborah Markiewicz, M.D., and Gerald E. Hanks, M.D., *International Journal of Radiation: Oncology, Biology, Physics*, vol. 20 (1991), pp. 153–167.

2. Letter to Dr. Seymour C. Nash, 1 Sept. 1992.

Chapter 10

1. In the four years since my TURP this number has declined markedly due to developments with other treatments for BPH: medicines, lasers, incision, even balloons.

2. For a blood coagulation test, a lab tech made a small cut in my arm, blotting it periodically until it dried. Coagulation time: six minutes. Was this good? Bad? About average, she said.

3. Some hospitals ask TURP patients to store up to two units of their own blood in anticipation of possible blood loss during the operation. A unit is slightly less than a pint. Since you can give up no more than one unit of blood a week, the advance time wasn't available. Dr. Nash didn't think it would be necessary, anyway, but if it were, I'd rather get my own back. Dr. Nash prefers the patient's own blood on standby for a radical prostatectomy but hasn't needed any for a TURP in years.

4. Not often, a patient might also experience some urgency of urination and/or some dribbling of urine, or could confront an inability to void altogether.

5. Heavy Medicare operating costs obviously, I thought, are increased by complicated and redundant handling costs. Hospital bills frequently are impossible to understand. About 30 percent of Medicare costs go to insurance carriers and others who pick up and put down pieces of paper. Various procedures are assigned a cost and if the doctor or hospital charges more than that, either you pay it or the hospital has to try to collect. Frequently, it cannot. So, those who can pay do so for themselves and also for those who cannot, or won't. Yet, for many pharmaceuticals, Medicare pays whatever's charged. It is a very expensive and inconsistent system, hardly congruent with our vaunted Yankee economic and managerial talents.

Chapter 11

1. A block cutter follows the configuration onto styrofoam from which a mold is created. A low melting point alloy, known as "cerrobend" or "osterloy," is poured into the mold to form the final block. So here in the hospital they're making molds, melting metal, pouring it into molds, trimming the casting and affixing it to a plexiglass plate, all operations by people with at least three years' specialized training, frequently much more.

2. This is a subject of continuing debate between surgeons and radiologists. The latter point out that surgery frequently treats patients who are healthier, who possess a longer life expectancy going into treatment, and who present less advanced cancers than the general run of radiation patients. The Cancer Society information office said it knew of no studies comparing surgery and radiation disease-free survival statistics on a stage-by-stage basis. But, then, the neutral Society may have been ducking an interdisciplinary bullet. There are newer reports from various cancer treatment centers involving a limited number of patients that uphold the surgeons' assertions. However, a stern statistician might argue with them. There are also reported in progress at this writing some NCI (National Cancer Institute) trials addressing radiation versus surgery for fifteen-year disease-free survival figures. I reiterate that fifteen-year survival in this 1990s study means the men were treated with pre-1980 methods and skills. On the practical side, in their day-to-day care of patients, urologists and radiotherapists work closely together. They consult with each other regularly on patient progress. Indeed, as I write this, Drs. Nash and Toonkel are cooperating at Mt. Sinai hospital in studies of brachytherapy, the implantation of radioactive seeds, on a number of selected patients.

3. Stephen N. Rous, M.D., *The Prostate Book* (N.Y.: W. W. Norton, 1992); Ruben F. Gittes, M.D., "Carcinoma of the Prostate," *New England Journal of Medicine*, 24 January, 1991, pp. 236–245.

4. In radiation treatment follow-up, the PSA level may decline even more at eight and twelve months. Some reports I read gave 0.4 as the lowest level of detectability; others gave 0.2, even 0.1, depending on the standards of the particular test, but in these reports the follow-up was to radical prostatectomies after which the PSA drops far more swiftly than after radiation because the prostate itself is gone and, presumably, the cancer with it.

5. Some say the rate of rise is more critical than the level. One researcher regards 4.0 ng/ml as evidence of treatment failure, dictating a need for biopsies.

Chapter 12

1. Arthur T. Porter, M.D., and Jeffrey D. Forman, M.D., Wayne State University School of Medicine, "Prostate Brachytherapy: An Overview," paper presented at the conference Prostate Cancer Detection and Management Controversies in the 1990s, Nov. 6 and 7, 1992, available from the author. (Much of the information in this section is attributable to Dr. Porter and colleagues.)

2. John C. Blasko, M.D., Peter D. Grimm, M.D., and Haakon Ragde, M.D., Northwest Tumor Institute, Seattle, "Brachytherapy and Organ Preservation in the Management of Carcinoma of the Prostate," *Seminars in Radiation Oncology*, vol. 3, no. 4 (Oct. 1993), pp. 240–249.

3. Iodine-125 has a half-life of 90 days, palladium-103 a half-life of 17.5 days.

4. Stanley A. Brosnan, M.D., and Kenneth Tokita, M.D., "Transrectal Ultrasound-Guided Interstitial Radiation Therapy for Localized Prostate Cancer," *Urology*, vol. 38, no. 4 (Oct. 1991), pp. 372–376.

Chapter 13

1. Gary M. Onik, Jeffrey K. Cohen, and George D. Reyes, M.D.'s, Allegheny General Hospital; Pittsburgh, Pa.; Boris Rubinsky, Ph.D., University of California, Berkeley; Chang Zhoa Hua, and John Baust, Ph.D.'s, Cryomedical Sciences, Rockville, Md., "Transrectal Ultrasound-Guided Percutaneous Radical Cryosurgical Ablation of the Prostate," *Cancer*, vol. 72, no. 4 (August 15, 1993), pp. 1291–99.

2. Gerald W. Chodak, M.D., University of Chicago Prostate and Urology Center, Chicago, "Cryosurgery of the Prostate Revisited," ibid., pp. 1145–46.

Chapter 14

1. P. C. Walsh, M.D. "Radical Retropubic Prostatectomy with Reduced Morbidity: An Anatomic Approach." *NCI Monographs*, no. 7. Washington, D.C.: Government Printing Office, 1988:133–137. (NIH Publication no. 88-3005.)

2. *Update*, vol. 2, no. 1 (winter 1991).

3. A note on the anesthetic: an epidural affects all your pain nerve fibers; you are awake and retain your motor functions. A "spinal," on the other hand, knocks out everything in your lower body for one to five hours depending on the dose and medication.

4. This is a little side note: some of my friendly (who else?) readers during the composition of this book remonstrated with me that this section was "too technical" for the layman and urged me to simplify and shorten it. Even my wife, who has been a total participant in this consuming project, said, "You're going to have men going around

clutching themselves. Do they want to know this much about it?" I have tried to avoid a lot of medical jargon but feel that a man who's going to be cut open and have some of his innards removed would want every detail there is. It's amazing how swiftly we learn the technical stuff when we're involved. I didn't have a prostatectomy, of course, but I've talked with a host of guys who have, and they weren't reluctant to discuss it in detail. If I'm wrong, skip a few pages.

5. Studies by Drs. W. W. Scott and H. L. Boyd of the University of Rochester School of Medicine and Dentistry in 1969 revealed that patients with clinical C stage disease who were treated preoperatively by orchiectomy or synthetic estrogen (DES) therapy had ten-year postoperative survival rates, similar to those of carriers of B1 clinical nodules surgically treated at Johns Hopkins. Charles B. Brendler, M.D., associate professor of urology at Johns Hopkins, told an Orlando, Fla., seminar in November 1991 that a close study of the Scott/Boyd reports raised questions about their conclusions. Patients obviously were carefully selected, he said, and only forty-four were treated with their approach. Response to hormonal therapy was tested only by digital examinations, and patients had only minimal involvement of seminal vesicles. He questions the original staging of the patients and wonders whether some actually had organ-confined cancer to begin with. He raises the additional question of whether hormone therapy alone in such a selected population might have been equally as effective as the combination.

Analyzing recent studies, Dr. Brendler thinks it is possible that improved surgical techniques and not the adjuvant hormone therapy produced the favorable statistics. He stated: "There is no convincing evidence that 'downstaging' with hormonal therapy prior to radical prostatectomy is effective in clinical stage C cancer. . . . In my view, three to six months of hormonal therapy simply delays potentially curative treatment in men with clinically localized prostatic cancer and is of no benefit in men with clinical stage C disease."

Chapter 15

1. Many women are treated for various female problems with estrogen compounds. Since estrogen is natural to them, women do not seem to have the cardiovascular side effects men suffer.

2. LHRH drugs are used sometimes on women in fertility treatment, to increase estrogen.

3. Urologists cannot say definitely testosterone at any level causes prostate cancer, however, they have commented on the face that some internists prescribe it for men with hormone related problems. They disapprove vehemently of such administrations, especially in the absence of hard proof that no prostate cancer is present.

4. The Labrie et al., reports have drawn considerable negative comment. Dr. David Paulson, quoted previously, wrote without mentioning any names, that "those who emphasize this aspect of total androgen blockade interpret these previous studies with excessive enthusiasm." As a victim of PCa who doesn't know whether his cancer will recur before he is eventually run over by a truck or otherwise terminated, I kept digging for all the qualifications I could find bearing on the optimistic Labrie reports. I was reminded of my involvement years ago in high school debating when every time I turned over a new source of information it negated what I had just concluded was verifiable certainty. Part 2 of this book examines this scientific debate in more detail.

5. Flutamide can cause side effects, such as diarrhea, nausea and vomiting, breast enlargement, and other adverse reactions, including liver abnormalities, in a minority of patients. Overdoses can be harmful. For these reasons, some centers are experimenting with interrupting flutamide treatment after six months and checking results before resuming.

6. Ralph deVere White, M.D., et al., "Urinary Prostate Specific Antigen Levels: Role in Monitoring the Response of Prostate Cancer to Therapy," *Journal of Urology*, vol. 147 (1992), Mar., pp. 947–951.

Chapter 16

1. Horst Zincke, M.D., "Surgery, Adjuvant Tx Better Stage C Choice," *Urology Times*, April 1992, p. 24.

2. Wai S. Cheng, M.D., et al. (including Zincke), "Radical Prostatectomy for Pathologic Stage C Prostate Cancer: Influence of Pathologic Variables and Adjuvant Treatment on Disease Outcome," *Urology*, vol. 42, no. 3 Sept. 1993), pp. 283–291.

3. Curtis Mettlin, Ph.D., George W. Jones, M.D., Gerald P. Murphy, M.D., "Trends in Prostate Cancer Care in the United States, 1974–1990," *Ca: A Cancer Journal for Clinicians*, vol. 43, no. 2 (March/April 1993), pp. 83–91.

4. Robert P. Myers, M.D., et al., "Hormonal Treatment at Time of Radical Retropubic Prostatectomy for Stage D1 Prostate Cancer: Results of Long-Term Follow-up," *Journal of Urology*, vol. 147 (March 1992), pp. 910–915.

Chapter 17

1. Paul F. Schellhammer, M.D., et al., "Local Failure after Definitive Radiation or Surgical Therapy for Carcinoma of the Prostate and Options for Prevention and Therapy," *Urologic Clinics of North America*, vol. 18, no. 3 (Aug. 1991).

2. Dr. von Eschenbach kindly sent us an advance copy of the abstract of his paper with the knowledge that this book would not be circulated until after the meeting. Participating with him in the report were Drs. David A. Swanson, R. Joseph Babaian, Colin P. N. Dinney, and Robert B. Evans.

3. Malcolm A. Bagshaw, M.D., in *Us Too*, the newsletter of the Prostate Cancer Support Group, vol. 1, no. 4 (August/September 1993). Dr. Bagshaw is the Henry S. Kaplan and Harry Lebeson Professor in Cancer Biology, emeritus, Dept. of Radiation Oncology, Division of Radiation Therapy, Stanford University Medical Center, Calif.

4. Judd D. Moul, M.D., David F. Paulson, M.D., Duke University Medical Center, "The Role of Radical Surgery in the Management of Radiation Recurrent and Large Volume Prostate Cancer," *Cancer*, vol. 68 (1991).

5. Irving D. Kaplan, M.D., and Malcolm A. Bagshaw, M.D., Stanford University Medical Center, "Serum Prostate-specific Antigen after Post-Prostatectomy Radiotherapy," *Urology*, vol. 39, no. 5 (May 1992).

6. R. Meier, M.D., et al., Palo Alto Medical Center, UCLA, "Postoperative Radiation Therapy after Radical Prostatectomy for Prostate Carcinoma Cancer, 1992," briefed in *Yearbook of Urology 1993*, Mosby–Year Book, Inc., St. Louis, Mo.

7. A. Stein, M.D., J. B. deKernion, M.D., F. Dorey, M.D., University of California at Los Angeles; R. B. Smith, M.D., Jonsson Comprehensive Cancer Center, Los

Angeles, "Adjuvant Radiotherapy in Patients Post-Radical Prostatectomy with Tumor Extending through Capsule or Positive Seminal Vesicles," *Urology,* Jan. 1992; briefed in *Yearbook of Urology 1993,* Mosby–Yearbook Inc., St. Louis, Mo.

8. David F. Paulson, M.D., professor and chief, division of urologic surgery, Duke University Medical Center, Durham, N.C., "Margin Positive Residual after Radical Prostatectomy," in *Advances in Urology,* 1992, ed. B. Lytton, M.D. (St. Louis, Mo.: Mosby).

9. Horst Zincke, M.D., Mayo Clinic, Rochester, Mn., letter to Seymour Nash, M.D., Miami, Sept. 1, 1992.

10. Jean B. deKernion, M.D., Chief of the Division of Urology, UCLA School of Medicine, letter to Seymour Nash, M.D., Aug. 31, 1992.

11. William R. Fair, M.D., Chief, Urologic Surgery, Memorial Sloan-Kettering Cancer Center, N.Y., letter to Seymour Nash, M.D., Sept. 10, 1992.

12. Wai S. Cheng, M.D., et al., "Radical Prostatectomy for Pathologic Stage C Prostate Cancer: Influence of Pathologic Variables and Adjuvant Treatment on Disease Outcome," *Urology,* vol. 42, no. 3 (Sept. 1993), pp. 283–291.

Chapter 18

1. Dr. Schover, who spoke to me at the National Conference on Prostate Cancer held in San Francisco in 1992, recommends an American Cancer Society booklet, *Sexuality and Cancer, for the Man with Cancer and His Partner,* as a good introduction to posttherapy sex adjustment. I refer you to two of her essays: "Sexual Rehabilitation after Treatment for Prostate Cancer," *Cancer,* vol. 71, suppl. (1993), pp. 1024–1030; and her chapter in a recently revised textbook: L. R. Schover, W. S. Schain, and D. K. Montague, "Sexual Problems of Patients with Cancer," in V. T. DeVita, S. Hellman, and S. A. Rosenberg, eds., *Cancer: Principles and Practice of Oncology,* 3d ed. (Philadelphia: J. B. Lippincott, 1989), pp. 2206–2225.

2. Among others, the Geddings Osborn Sr. Foundation, 1246 Jones St., Augusta, Ga. 30901; and American Medical Systems Information Center, Minnetonka, Minn.

Chapter 19

1. This is a decision I had to make and I wish I had had this book, or something as thorough, to read before doing so.—SM

2. At some centers in the seventies and eighties you would have received routinely a pelvic lymph node dissection and open insertion of radioactive iodine-125 seeds. Today, if qualified, you would be offered a radical prostatectomy. The standards of treatment may change according to the leadership at various centers, what research they are doing, and what national protocols they are committed to. Sometimes, what's best for the patient may not fit their research patterns.

Chapter 20

1. The Mathews Foundation's address is 1010 Hurley Way, Suite 195, Sacramento, Calif. 95825, 916/567-1400.

2. The American Foundation for Urologic Disease (AFUD) is headquartered at

the same address as the physicians' organization, the American Urological Association, Inc., 1120 N. Charles St., Baltimore, Md. 21201.

3. Sympathetic doctors also point out that this is a time in a man's life when other significant changes are taking place; perhaps in his career, perhaps in sexual performance, perhaps in increased distance from his growing children or even perhaps in problems with his wife due to a difficult menopause on her part. If you want to delve into the mind's control over the body or relationships between emotions and health, the simple effect of age on bodily functions might be a good place to start.

Chapter 22

1. Ruben F. Gittes, M.D., review, "Carcinoma of the Prostate," *New England Journal of Medicine,* vol. 324, no. 4 (Jan. 24, 1991).

2. A Moon Pie, once almost a staple of Southern confectionary, consists of two slabs of chocolate-covered graham-cracker-like cake with a hearty layer of marshmallow in between, the total about the size of a skinny hamburger. Or you can get them in a doubled variety.

3. Wilhelm A. Bitterman, M.D., et al., "Environmental and Nutritional Factors Significantly Associated with Cancer of the Urinary Tract among Different Ethnic Groups," *Urologic Clinics of North America,* vol. 18, no. 1 (August 1993), pp. 501–508.

4. Brian E. Henderson, M.D., "Summary Report of the Sixth Symposium on Cancer Registries and Epidemiology in the Pacific Basin," *Journal of the National Cancer Institute,* vol. 82, no. 14 (July 18, 1990), pp. 1186–1190.

5. Ann W. Hsing et al., "Serologic Precursors of Cancer, Retinoil, Carotenoids, and Tocopherol and Risk of Prostate Cancer," *Journal of the National Cancer Institute,* vol. 82, no. 11 (June 6, 1990), pp. 941–945.

6. Edward Giovannucci, M.D., et al., "A Prospective Study of Dietary Fat and Risk of Prostate Cancer," *Journal of the National Cancer Institute,* vol. 85, no. 19 (Oct. 6, 1993); Kenneth J. Pienta, M.D., and Peggy S. Esper, editorial, "Is Dietary Fat a Risk Factor for Prostate Cancer?" *Journal of the National Cancer Institute,* vol. 85, no. 19 (Oct. 6, 1993), pp. 1538–1539.

7. *Wall Street Journal,* Feb. 16, 1994, p. B5.

8. Monroe Greenberger, M.D., and Mary-Ellen Siegel, M.S.W., *What Every Man Should Know about His Prostate,* rev. ed. (N.Y.: Walker, 1988).

9. There is a high concentration of zinc in seminal fluid and the prostate but there is some question whether zinc taken orally, separately, rather than in zinc-rich foods, gets to the prostate.

Chapter 23

1. I could not help but apply a reporter's skepticism to this enormous figure, so I asked Dr. Labrie where he got it. He started with the world census of males, applied the percentages of prostate cancer among them, using only half of the U.S. and Western Europe percentages for the remainder of the world. The western world has double the rate of everywhere else, if claiming superlatives pleases your ego. Of course, many of these victims will never be diagnosed or treated. They may die of their cancer or succumb to something else before the cancer gets them.

Chapter 26

1. Personal interview with S. Meyer. See Thomas A. Stamey, M.D., "Prostate Specific Antigen—1990 Overview," *Report on the Fifth Annual Symposium: Transrectal Ultrasound in the Diagnosis and Management of Prostate Cancer, Sept. 14–15, 1990,* (American Urological Association Office of Education, 1991), pp. 54–68.

2. John N. Kabalin, M.D., Stanford University School of Medicine, "Stage A Prostate Cancer Today" (editorial), *Journal of Urology,* vol. 150 (Nov. 1993), pp. 1749–1750.

3. Anthony V. D'Amico, M.D., and Gerald E. Hanks, M.D., Fox Chase Cancer Center, Philadelphia, Pa., "Linear Regressive Analysis Using Prostate-Specific Antigen Doubling Time for Predicting Tumor Biology and Clinical Outcome in Prostate Cancer," *Cancer,* vol. 72, no. 9 (Nov. 1, 1993), pp. 2638–2643.

Chapter 27

1. G. E. Hanks, M.D., et al., "A Ten Year Follow-up of 682 Patients Treated for Prostate Cancer with Radiation Therapy in the U.S.," *International Journal of Radiation: Oncology, Biology, Physics,* vol. 13, pp. 449–505.

2. Irving D. Kaplan, M.D., et al., Stanford School of Medicine, "The Importance of Local Control in the Treatment of Prostatic Cancer," *Journal of Urology,* vol. 147, pp. 917–921 (March 1992).

Chapter 28

1. Explains Gary Ayers, M.D., radiation therapist at Northside Hospital, Atlanta, Ga., in a letter to Sylvan Meyer, Dec. 31, 1991: in linear accelerator machines, "basically electrons are taken from a standard electrical current and accelerated through a magnetic tunnel to high speeds. These electrons strike a special metal target. The interaction of the high speed electrons with the special metal target produces x-rays."

2. Drs. Barry E. Epstein and Gerald E. Hanks, "Prostate Cancer: Evaluation and Radiotherapeutic Management," *Ca—A Cancer Journal for Clinicians,* vol. 42, no. 4 (July/August 1992), pp. 223–240.

Chapter 29

1. Letter March 30, 1992, from Dr. John C. Blasko, director, Northwest Tumor Institute, to Dr. Seymour C. Nash.

2. Letter April 1, 1992, from Dr. Stanley A. Brosman, Santa Monica, Calif., Urologic Medical Group, to Dr. Seymour C. Nash.

Chapter 30

1. James M. Kozlowski, William J. Ellis, and John T. Grayhack, "Advanced Prostate Carcinoma: Early vs. Late Endocrine Therapy," *Urologic Clinics of North America,* vol. 18, no. 1 (Feb. 1991), pp. 15–24.

2. David F. Paulson, M.D., "Margin Positive Residual after Radical Prostatectomy: Value of Adjunctive Therapy," in *Advances in Urology,* ed. B. Lytton, M.D. (St. Louis: Mosby).

Chapter 31

1. Horst Zincke, M.D., "Radical Prostatectomy and Exenterative Procedures for Local Failure after Radiotherapy with Curative Intent; Comparison of Outcomes," *Journal of Urology,* March 1992, vol. 174, pp. 894–899.

2. For more details, see David F. Paulson, M.D., "Margin Positive Residual after Radical Prostatectomy: Value of Adjunctive Therapy," in *Advances in Urology,* ed. B. Lytton, M.D. (St. Louis: Mosby, 1992).

3. B. R. Cassileth, M.D., *Quality of Life and Psychosocial Status in Stage D Prostate Cancer,* corporation reprint available from Gerard T. Kennealey, M.D., Director of Oncology Research, ICI Pharmaceuticals, Concord Pike and Murphy Road, Wilmington, Del. 19897.

Chapter 32

1. Howard Scher, M.D., "Prostatic Cancer: Where Do We Go from Here?" *Current Opinion in Oncology,* 1991, vol. 3, pp. 568–574.

2. Dr. Scher's figures include men of all ages. Mortality is higher in older men. That is why a ten-year life expectancy should be a prerequisite for surgery.

3. Willet F. Whitmore, Jr., M.D., "Management of Clinically Localized Prostatic Cancer: An Unresolved Problem," *Journal of the American Medical Association,* vol. 269, no. 20 (May 16, 1993), pp. 2676–2677.

4. Fernand Labrie, M.D., et al., "Serum Prostate Specific Antigen as a Pre-Screening Test for Prostate Cancer," *Journal of Urology,* vol. 147 (March 1991), pp. 846–852.

Chapter 33

1. See *Scientific American,* Feb. 1992.

Bibliography

Adolfsson, Jan, M.D.; Gunnar Steineck, M.D.; and Willet Whitmore, Jr.,
M.D. "Recent Results of Management of Palpable Clinically Localized Prostate Cancer," *Cancer*, vol. 72, no. 2 (July 15, 1993),
pp. 310–322.

Andriole, Gerald L., M.D., and William J. Catalona, M.D., guest editors,
Urologic Clinics of North America, vol. 18, no. 1 (Feb. 1991): *Advanced
Prostatic Carcinoma.*

Anscher, Mitchell S., M.D., and Leonard R. Prosnitz, M.D. "Prognostic
Significance of Extent of Nodal Involvement in Stage D1 Prostate
Cancer Treated with Radiotherapy." *Urology*, vol. 39, no. 1 (Jan.
1992), pp. 39–43.

Bagshaw, Malcolm A., M.D. "Local Recurrence of Prostate Cancer after
Radiotherapy." *Us Too*, vol. 1, no. 4 (Aug./Sept. 1993) (Prostate Cancer Support Group international newsletter), pp. 1, 3.

Barry, Michael D., M.D. "Prostate Surgery: Risk, Benefit, Uncertainty,"
Medical Forum in *Harvard Medical School Health Letter*, June 1989,
pp. 5–7.

Benson, George S., M.D. "Mechanisms of Penile Erection." *Investigative
Urology*, vol. 19, no. 2 (Sept. 1981), pp. 65–69.

Bilhartz, David L., M.D.; D. J. Tindall, Ph.D.; and J. E. Oesterling, M.D.
"Prostate-Specific Antigen and Prostatic Acid Phosphatase: Bio-
molecular and Physiologic Characteristics." *Urology*, vol. 38, no. 2
(Aug. 1991), pp. 95–102.

Bitterman, Wilhelm A., M.D., et al. "Environmental and Nutritional Factors Significantly Associated with Cancer of the Urinary Tract among
Different Ethnic Groups." *Urologic Clinics of North America*, vol. 18,
no. 3 (Aug. 1991), pp. 501–508.

Blasko, John C., M.D.; Peter D. Grimm, M.D.; and Haakon Ragde, M.D.
"Brachytherapy and Organ Preservation in the Management of Carci-
noma of the Prostate." *Seminars in Radiation Oncology*, vol. 3, no. 4
(Oct. 1993), pp. 240–249.

Blasko, John C., M.D.; Haakon Ragde, M.D.; and Peter D. Grimm, M.D. "Transperineal Ultrasound-Guided Implantation of the Prostate: Morbidity and Complications." *Scandinavian Journal of Urology and Nephrology*, supplement no. 137, *Ultrasound in Urology*, Jorgen Kvist Kristenson, Niels Juul, and Soren Torp-Pederson, eds., pp. 113–118. Copenhagen, Denmark, 1991.

Bostwick, David G., M.D. "The Pathology of Early Prostate Cancer." *Ca—A Cancer Journal for Clinicians*, vol. 39, no. 6 (Nov./Dec. 1989), pp. 376–393.

Brawer, Michael K., M.D. "Predictors of Pathologic State in Prostatic Carcinoma: The Role of Neovascularity." *Cancer*, vol. 73, no. 3 (Feb. 1, 1994), pp. 678–687.

Brawer, Michael K., M.D., and Paul H. Lange, M.D. "Prostate-Specific Antigen and Premalignant Change: Implications for Early Detection." *Ca—A Cancer Journal for Clinicians*, vol. 39, no. 6 (Nov./Dec. 1989), pp. 361–375.

Brendler, Charles B., M.D. *Role of Radiotherapy in Localized Prostate Cancer*. Report on seminar: Carcinoma of the Prostate, Orlando, Fla., Nov. 16, 1991. American Urological Association Office of Education.

Brosnan, Stanley A., M.D., and Kenneth Tokita, M.D. "Transrectal Ultrasound-Guided Interstitial Radiation Therapy for Localized Prostate Cancer." *Urology*, vol. 38, no. 4 (Oct. 1991), pp. 372–376.

Brown, Elizabeth, M.D. "Balloon Dilation Offers Option for Prostate Procedure." *American Medical News*, Sept. 1, 1989.

Cancer Facts and Figures—1992. Atlanta: American Cancer Society, 1992.

Cancer of the Prostate. Research report, National Cancer Institute, NIH Publ. No. 91-528, Sept. 1990.

Cancer, vol. 70, no. 1 (July 1992), supplement: *American Cancer Society / American Urological Association International Workshop of Prostatic Cancer and Hyperplasia, Sea Island, Georgia, Oct. 26–29, 1991*.

Carter, H. Ballentine, M.D., Jay D. Pearson, M.D., et al. "Longitudinal Evaluation of Prostate-Specific Antigen Levels in Men with and without Prostate Disease." *Journal of the American Medical Association*, vol. 267, no. 16 (Apr. 22/29, 1992).

Cassileth, Barrie R., Ph.D., et al. "Patient's Choice of Treatment in Stage D Prostate Cancer." Supplement to *Urology*, vol. 33, no. 5 (May 1989), pp. 57–62.

Cassileth, Barrie R., Ph.D., M. S. Soloway, M.D., et al. "Quality of Life and Psychosocial Status in Stage D Prostate Cancer." *Quality of Life Research*, vol. 1 (1992), pp. 323–330. Reprints available from Gerard T. Kennealey, M.D., Director of Oncology Research, ICI Pharmaceuticals, Concord Pike and Murphy Road, Wilmington, DE 19897.

Catalona, Wm. J., M.D. *Prostate Cancer.* Orlando, Fla.: Grune and Stratton, 1984.

―――. "PSA and the Detection of Prostate Cancer." *Journal of the American Medical Association,* vol. 271, no. 3 (Jan. 19, 1994), p. 192.

Catalona, Wm. J., M.D., and W. W. Scott, M.D. "Carcinoma of the Prostate." *Campbell's Urology,* 5th ed., chap. 32. Philadelphia: W. B. Saunders, 1986.

Catalona, Wm. J., M.D., et al. "Measurement of Prostate-Specific Antigen in Serum as a Screening Test for Prostate Cancer." *New England Journal of Medicine,* vol. 324, no. 17 (Apr. 25, 1991), pp. 1156–1161.

Chemotherapy and You: A Guide to Self-Help during Treatment. U.S. Dept. of Health and Human Services, Public Health Service, National Institutes of Health, National Cancer Institute, NIH Publication No. 88-136.

Cheng, Wai S., M.D., et al. "Radical Prostatectomy for Pathologic Stage C Prostate Cancer: Influence of Pathologic Variables and Adjuvant Treatment on Disease Outcome." *Urology,* vol. 42, no. 3 (Sept. 1993), pp. 283–291.

Chodak, Gerald W., M.D. "Cryosurgery of the Prostate Revisited" (editorial). *Cancer,* vol. 72, no. 4 (Aug. 15, 1993), pp. 1145–1146.

Chodak, Gerald W., M.D., et al. "Effect of External Beam Radiation Therapy on Serum Prostate Specific Antigen." *Urology,* vol. 35, no. 4 (Apr. 1990), pp. 288–294.

Chodak, Gerald W., M.D., et al. "Results of Conservative Management of Clinically Localized Prostate Cancer." *New England Journal of Medicine,* vol. 330, no. 4 (Jan. 27, 1994), pp. 242–248.

Cooner, William H., M.D. "Endorectal Ultrasonography Beneficial in Monitoring Prostate Cancer after Definitive Therapy." *A.U.A. Today,* vol. 4, no. 9 (Sept. 1991), p. 9.

Cotton, Paul. "Case for Prostate Therapy Wanes despite More Treatment Options" (editorial). *Journal of the American Medical Association,* vol. 266, no. 4 (July 24, 1991), pp. 459–460.

Cousins, Norman. *Anatomy of an Illness as Perceived by the Patients: Reflections of Healing and Regeneration.* New York: Bantam Books, 1981.

―――. *Head First.* New York: Penguin Books USA, 1989.

Crawford, E. David, M.D. "Prostate Cancer Awareness Week Data Suggest PSA plus DRE Most Effective Screening Method." *A.U.A. Today,* vol. 4, no. 9 (Sept. 1991), p. 8.

Cunningham, Chet. *Your Prostate: What Every Man over Forty Needs to Know . . . Now!* Leucadia, Cal.: United Research Publishers, 1990.

D'Amico, Anthony V., M.D., and Gerald E. Hanks, M.D. "Linear Regressive Analysis Using Prostate-Specific Antigen Doubling Time for Predicting Tumor Biology and Clinical Outcome in Prostate Cancer." *Cancer*, vol. 72, no. 9 (Nov. 1, 1993), pp. 2638–2643.

Davidson, Nancy E., M.D. "Tamoxifen—Panacea or Pandora's Box?" *New England Journal of Medicine*, vol. 326, no. 13 (Mar. 26, 1992), pp. 885–886.

Dawson, Nancy A., M.D., et al. "A Pilot Trial of Chemohormonal Therapy for Metastatic Prostate Carcinoma." *Cancer*, vol. 69, no. 1 (Jan. 1, 1992), pp. 213–217.

Doornbos, J. Frederick, M.D., et al. "Results of Radical Perineal Prostatectomy with Adjuvant Brachytherapy." *Radiology*, vol. 184, no. 2 (Aug. 1992), pp. 333–339.

Dowling, Robert A., M.D.; C. Humberto Carrasco, M.D.; and R. Joseph Babaian, M.D. "Percutaneous Urinary Diversion in Patients with Hormone-Refractory Prostate Cancer." *Urology*, vol. 38, no. 2 (Feb. 1991), pp. 89–91.

Doyle, G. Mark, and James L. Mohler. "Prediction of Metastatic Potential of Aspirated Cells from the Dunning R-3327 Prostatic Adenocarcinoma Model." *Journal of Urology*, Mar. 1992 (vol. 147), pp. 756–759.

Drago, Joseph R., M.D. "The Role of New Modalities in the Early Detection and Diagnosis of Prostate Cancer." *Ca—A Cancer Journal for Clinicians*, vol. 39, no. 6 (Nov./Dec. 1989), pp. 326–336.

Drago, Joseph R., M.D., et al. "Radical Prostatectomy: OSU and Affiliated Hospitals' Experience, 1985–1989." *Urology*, vol. 39, no. 1 (Jan. 1992), pp. 44–47.

Drago, Joseph R., M.D., et al. "Localized Staging of Prostate Carcinoma: Comparison of Transrectal Ultrasound and Magnetic Resonance Imaging." *Urology*, vol. 35, no. 6 (June 1990), pp. 511–512.

Eisbruch, Avraham, M.D., et al. "Adjuvant Irradiation after Prostatectomy for Carcinoma of the Prostate with Positive Surgical Margins." *Cancer*, vol. 73, no. 2 (Jan. 15, 1994), pp. 384–387.

Ennis, Ronald D., M.D., and Richard E. Peschel, M.D. "Radiation Therapy for Prostate Cancer, Long-Term Results and Implications for Future Advances." *Cancer*, vol. 72, no. 9 (Nov. 1, 1993), pp. 2644–2649.

Epstein, Jonathan I., M.D. "The Prostate and Seminal Vesicles." Chapter 41 of *Diagnostic Surgical Pathology*, ed. Stephan S. Sternberg, pp. 1393–1417. N.Y.: Raven Press, 1989.

Epstein, Jonathan I., M.D.; Patrick C. Walsh, M.D.; Marné Carmichael;

and Charles B. Brendler, M.D. "Pathologic and Clinical Findings to Predict Tumor Extent of Nonpalpable (Stage T1c) Prostate Cancer." *Journal of the American Medical Association*, vol. 217, no. 5 (Feb. 2, 1994), pp. 368–374.

Fellows, G. J., et al. (Urological Cancer Working Party—Subgroup on Prostatic Cancer). "Treatment of Advanced Localised Prostatic Cancer by Orchiectomy, Radiotherapy, or Combined Treatment." *British Journal of Urology*, vol. 70 (1992), pp. 304–309.

Fleming, Craig, M.D., et al. "A Decision Analysis of Alternative Treatment Strategies for Clinically Localized Prostate Cancer." *Journal of the American Medical Association*, vol. 269, no. 20 (May 26, 1993), pp. 2650–2658.

Frazier, Harold A., II; Judith E. Robertson, C.T.R.; and David F. Paulson, M.D. "Does Radical Prostatectomy in the Presence of Positive Pelvic Lymph Nodes Enhance Survival?" Research paper from the Division of Urology, Cancer Center Database, Duke University Medical Center, Durham, N.C. (Research performed while Dr. Frazier was serving as a fellow in urologic oncology with funding from the U.S. Navy.)

Gaillard-Moguilewsky, Martine, Ph.D. "Pharmacology of Antiandrogens and Value of Combining Androgen Suppression with Antiandrogen Therapy." Supplement to *Urology*, vol. 38, no. 2 (Feb. 1991), pp. 5–11.

Gerber, Glenn S., M.D., et al. "Disease Specific Survival Following Routine Prostate Cancer Screening by Digital Rectal Examination." *Journal of the American Medical Association*, vol. 269, no. 1 (Jan. 6, 1993), pp. 61–64.

Gibbons, Robert P., M.D. "Localized Prostate Carcinoma: Surgical Management." *Cancer*, vol. 72, no. 10 (Nov. 15, 1993), pp. 2865–2872.

Gillenwater, Jay Y., M.D., and Stuart S. Howards, M.D., eds. *The Yearbook of Urology*. St. Louis: Mosby, 1993.

Giovannucci, Edward, M.D., et al. "A Prospective Study of Dietary Fat and Risk of Prostate Cancer." *Journal of the National Cancer Institute*, vol. 85, no. 19 (Oct. 6, 1993), pp. 1571–1579.

Giovannucci, Edward, M.D., et al. "A Prospective Cohort Study of Vasectomy and Prostate Cancer in U.S. Men." *Journal of the American Medical Association*, vol. 269, no. 7 (Feb. 17, 1993), pp. 873–882.

Gittes, Ruben F., M.D. "Carcinoma of the Prostate" (ten-year summary). *New England Journal of Medicine*, vol. 324, no. 4 (Jan. 24, 1991), pp. 236–245.

Gomella, Leonard G., M.D., and John J. Fried. *Recovering from Prostate Cancer: A Doctor's Guide for Patients and Their Loved Ones*. New York: Harper Paperbacks, 1993.

Grayhack, John T., ed. See *Journal of Urology*, special issues.

Greenberger, Monroe, M.D., and Mary-Ellen Siegel, M.S.W. *What Every Man Should Know about His Prostate*, rev. ed. New York: Walker, 1988.

Hammarsten, Jan, and Klas Lindquist. "Suprapubic Catheter Following Transurethral Resection of the Prostate: A Way to Decrease the Number of Urethral Strictures and Improve the Outcome of Operations." *Journal of Urology*, vol. 147 (Mar. 1992), pp. 648–52.

Hanks, G. E., M.D. "External-Beam Radiation Therapy for Clinically Localized Prostate Cancer." *NCI Monographs*, no. 7, *NIH Consensus Development Conference on the Management of Clinically Localized Prostate Cancer* (1988), pp. 75–84.

Hanks, G. E., M.D., et al. "Outcome for Lymph Node Dissection T-1b, T-2 (A-2, B) Prostate Cancer Treated with External Beam Radiation Therapy in RTOG 77-06." *International Journal of Radiation: Oncology, Biology, Physics*, vol. 21 (1991), pp. 1099–1103.

Hanks, G. E., M.D., et al. "A Ten Year Follow-up of 682 Patients Treated for Prostate Cancer with Radiation Therapy in the U.S." *International Journal of Radiation: Oncology, Biology, Physics*, vol. 13 (Nov. 1987), pp. 499–505.

Henderson, Brian E., M.D. "Summary Report of the Sixth Symposium on Cancer Registries and Epidemiology in the Pacific Basin." *Journal of the National Cancer Institute*, vol. 82, no. 14 (July 18, 1990), pp. 1186–1190.

Howards, Stuart S., M.D., and Herbert B. Peterson, M.D. "Vasectomy and Prostate Cancer: Chance, Bias, or a Causal Relationship" (editorial). *Journal of the American Medical Association*, vol. 269, no. 7 (Feb. 17, 1993), pp. 913–914.

Hsing, Ann W., et al. "Serologic Precursors of Cancer: Retinol, Carotenoids, and Tocopherol and Risk of Prostate Cancer." *Journal of the National Cancer Institute*, vol. 82, no. 11 (June 6, 1990), pp. 941–946.

Huben, Robert P., M.D., and Gerald P. Murphy, M.D. "Prostate Cancer: An Update." American Cancer Society Professional Education Publication, reprinted from *Ca—A Cancer Journal for Clinicians*, vol. 36 (1986), pp. 274–292.

Jenner, Seth P., et al. "The Risk of Dying of Prostate Cancer in Patients with Clinically Localized Disease." *Journal of Urology*, vol. 146 (Oct. 1991), pp. 1040–1045.

Johansson, Jan-Erik, M.D., Ph.D., et al. "High Ten-Year Survival Rate in Patients with Early, Untreated Prostatic Cancer." *Journal of the American Medical Association*, vol. 267, no. 16 (Apr. 22/29, 1992), pp. 2191–2196.

Journal of Urology, special issue: *BPH/Obstruction,* vol. 150, no. 5, part 2 of 2 (Nov. 1993), John T. Greyhack, ed.

Journal of Urology, special issue: *Prostate Carcinoma,* vol. 147, no. 3, part 2 of 2 (Mar. 1992), John T. Greyhack, ed.

Kahn, Zafar, M.D.; Maria Mieza, M.D.; Perry Starer, M.D.; and Vinod K. Singh, M.D. "Post-Prostatectomy Incontinence: A Urodynamic and Fluoroscopic Point of View." *Urology,* vol. 38, no. 5 (Nov. 1991), pp. 483–488.

Kane, Robert A., M.D., et al. "Prostate Specific Antigen Levels in 1,695 Men without Evidence of Prostate Cancer: Findings of the American Cancer Society National Prostate Cancer Detection Project, A Multi-center, Multidisciplinary Trial." *Cancer,* vol. 59, no. 5 (Mar. 1992), pp. 1201–1207.

Kaplan, Irving D., M.D., and Malcolm A. Bagshaw, M.D. "Serum Prostate-Specific Antigen after Post-Prostatectomy Radiotherapy." *Urology,* vol. 39, no. 5 (May 1992), pp. 401–406.

Killian, Carl S., M.D., et al. "Prognostic Importance of Prostate-Specific Antigen for Monitoring Patients with Stages B2 to D1 Prostate Cancer." *Cancer Research,* vol. 45 (Feb. 1985), pp. 886–891.

Kynaston, H. G., et al. "Radiotherapy for Palliation of Locally Advanced Prostatic Carcinoma." *British Journal of Urology,* vol. 66, no. 5 (Nov. 1990), pp. 515–517.

Labrie, Fernand, M.D., Ph.D. "Endocrine Therapy for Prostate Cancer." *Endocrinology and Metabolism Clinics of North America,* vol. 20, no. 4 (Dec. 1991), pp. 845–872.

Labrie, Fernand, M.D., Ph.D., André Dupont, M.D., and Alain Belanger, M.D. "Combined Therapy with an LHRH Agonist and a Pure Anti-androgen in Prostate Cancer." In *Andrology: Male Fertility and Sterility,* ed. John D. Paulson, pp. 39–55. Orlando, Fla.: Harcourt Brace Jovanovich, 1986.

———. "Complete Androgen Blockade for the Treatment of Prostate Cancer." In *Important Advances in Oncology,* ed. V. T. Devita, Jr., S. Hellman, and S. A. Rosenberg, p. 193. Philadelphia, Pa.: Lippincott, 1985.

Labrie, Fernand, M.D., Ph.D., et al. "Serum Prostate Specific Antigen as Pre-Screening Test for Prostate Cancer." *Journal of Urology,* vol. 147 (Mar. 1992), pp. 846–852.

Labrie, Fernand, M.D., Ph.D., et al. "Combination Therapy for Prostate Cancer: Endocrine and Biological Basis of Its Choice as New Standard First Line Therapy." Paper presented at American Cancer Society National Conference on Prostate Cancer, San Francisco, Calif.,

Feb. 13–15, 1992. Reprints: CHUL Research Center, 2705 Laurier Blvd., Quebec, G1V 4G2, Canada.

Laliberte, Richard. "When Cancer Hits below the Belt," part 3 of 3. *Men's Confidential* (newsletter of *Prevention* and *Men's Health* magazines), vol. 9, no. 3 (Mar. 1994), pp. 11–12.

Lange, Paul H., M.D. "The Next Era for Prostate Cancer: Controlled Clinical Trials." *Journal of the American Medical Association,* vol. 269, no. 1 (Jan. 6, 1993), pp. 94–95.

Lenninger, J. Michael. "Balloon Therapy Tested for Enlarged Prostate." *The Center* (newsletter of the University of Florida Health Science Center), vol. 27, no. 1 (fall 1990), p. 7.

Lepor, Herbert, M.D. "Can BPH Be Treated with Drugs?" *Contemporary Urology,* June/July 1989, pp. 15–23.

Lerner, Seth P., M.D., et al. "The Risk of Dying of Prostate Cancer in Patients with Clinically Localized Disease." *Journal of Urology,* Oct. 1991 (vol. 146), pp. 1040–1045.

Leslie, Stephen W., M.D. *Impotence: Current Diagnosis and Treatment.* Geddings Osborn Sr. Foundation publication. Lorain, Ohio, Sept. 1990.

Lilley, Linda L., R.N., M.S. "Impact of Radiation on Prostate Cancer: Here's How to Help Patients Cope with the Side Effects of Treatment for the No. 1 Cancer in Men." *Geriatric Nursing,* July/August 1991, pp. 174–176.

Lu-Yao, Grace L., Ph.D., et al. "An Assessment of Radical Prostatectomy: Time Trends, Geographic Variation, and Outcomes." *Journal of the American Medical Association,* vol. 269, no. 20 (May 26, 1993), pp. 2633–2636.

Mann, Charles C. "The Prostate Cancer Dilemma." *Atlantic Monthly,* Nov. 1993, pp. 102–118.

Markiewicz, Deborah, M.D., and Gerald E. Hanks, M.D. "Therapeutic Options in the Management of Incidental Carcinoma of the Prostate." *International Journal of Radiation: Oncology, Biology, Physics,* vol. 20 (1991), pp. 153–167.

Mayo Health Clinic Clinical Update, vol. 7, no. 4 (summer 1991). *New Treatment Options for Benign Prostate Hypertrophy.*

McCullough, David L., M.D., et al. "Transurethral Balloon Dilation of the Prostate: An Alternative to Transurethral Resection?" *A.U.A. Today,* Jan. 1990.

McLeod, David G., M.D., et al. "Controversies in the Treatment of Metastatic Prostate Cancer." *Cancer* (supplement), vol. 70, no. 1 (July 1, 1992), pp. 324–328.

Mettlin, Curtis, Ph.D.; George W. Jones, M.D.; and Gerald P. Murphy, M.D. "Trends in Prostate Cancer Care in the United States 1974–1990: Observations from the Patient Care Evaluation Studies of the American College of Surgeons Commission on Cancer." *Ca—A Cancer Journal for Clinicians*, vol. 43, no. 2 (Mar./Apr. 1993), pp. 83–91.

Milroy, Evan. "Clinical Overview of Prazosin in the Treatment of Prostatic Obstruction." *Urology International*, vol. 45 (supplement 1), pp. 1–3.

Moon, Timothy D., M.D., and Sanda Clejan, M.D. "Prostate Cancer Screening in Younger Men: Prostate-Specific Antigen and Public Awareness." *Urology*, vol. 38, no. 3 (Sept. 1991), pp. 216–219.

Moul, Judd W., M.D., and David F. Paulson, M.D. "The Role of Radical Surgery in the Management of Radiation Recurrent and Large Volume Prostate Cancer." *Cancer*, vol. 68, no. 6 (Sept. 15, 1991), pp. 1265–1271.

Murphy, Gerald P., M.D. "Progress against Prostate Cancer." In *Prostate Cancer: Pathology, Detection, and Diagnosis*. American Cancer Society Professional Education Publication. Atlanta: ACS, 1990. Reprinted from *Ca—A Cancer Journal for Clinicians*, vol. 39 (1989), pp. 325–393.

———, ed. *Cancer Statistics, 1991*. Reprint from *Ca—A Cancer Journal for Clinicians*, vol. 1, no. 1 (Jan./Feb. 1991).

National Cancer Institute. *Cancer of the Prostate: Research Report*. NIH Publication No. 91-528, Sept. 1990.

———. *Eating Hints: Tips and Recipes for Better Nutrition during Cancer Treatment*. U.S. Dept. of Health and Human Services, Public Health Service, NIH Publication No. 91-2079, Dec. 1990.

National Institute of Health Consensus Development Conference Statement on the Management of Clinically Localized Prostate Cancer, June 15–17, 1987. No. 7 of *National Cancer Institute Monographs*. 1988.

Nativ, Ofer, M.D., et al. "Stage C Prostatic Adenocarcinoma: Flow Cytometric Nuclear DNA Ploidy Analysis." *Mayo Clinic Proceedings*, vol. 64, no. 8 (Aug. 1989), pp. 911–919.

Newsweek. August 5, 1991; cancer article, p. 48.

Oesterling, Joseph E., M.D. "PSA Leads the Way for Detecting and Following Prostate Cancer." *Contemporary Urology*, Feb. 1993, pp. 60–81.

———. Interview in *Urology Times*. See Weems, W. Lamar.

Oesterling, Joseph E., M.D.; Sandra K. Martin, R.N.; et al. "The Use of Prostate-Specific Antigen in Staging Patients with Newly Diagnosed Prostate Cancer." *Journal of the American Medical Association*, vol. 269, no. 1 (Jan. 6, 1993), pp. 57–60.

Onik, Gary M., M.D.; Jeffrey K. Cohen, M.D.; George D. Reyes, M.D.;

Boris Rubinsky, Ph.D.; Zhoa Hua Chang, Ph.D.; and John Baust, Ph.D. "Transrectal Ultrasound-Guided Percutaneous Radical Cryosurgical Ablation of the Prostate." *Cancer,* vol. 72, no. 4 (Aug. 15, 1993), pp. 1291–1298.

Partin, Alan W., M.D., Ph.D.; Gary D. Steinberg, M.D.; et al. "Use of Nuclear Morphometry, Gleason Histologic Scoring, Clinical Stage, and Age to Predict Disease-Free Survival among Patients with Prostate Cancer." *Cancer,* vol. 70, no. 1 (July 1, 1992), pp. 161–168.

Paulson, David F., M.D. "Margin Positive Residual after Radical Prostatectomy: Value of Adjunctive Therapy." *Advances in Urology,* 1992, ed. B. Lytton, M.D. St. Louis: Mosby.

Paulson, David F., M.D.; Judd W. Moul, M.D.; and Philip J. Walther, M.D. "Radical Prostatectomy for Clinical Stage T1-2N0M0 Prostatic Adenocarcinoma: Long Term Results." *Journal of Urology,* vol. 144 (Nov. 1990), pp. 1180–1184.

Perez, C. A., M. V. Pilepich, D. Garcia, et al. "Definitive Radiation Therapy in Carcinoma of the Prostate Localized to the Pelvis: Experience of the Mallinckrodt Institute of Radiology." *NCI Monographs,* no. 7 (1988), pp. 85–94.

Peschel, Richard E., M.D., Ph.D. "External Beam vs. Interstitial Implant Therapy for Prostate Cancer: A Review." *Endocurie Therapy/Hyperthermia Oncology,* July/Oct. 1990 (vol. 6), pp. 231–237.

Pilepich, M. V., M.D., et al. "Definitive Radiotherapy in Resectable (Stage A2 and B) Carcinoma of the Prostate—Results of a Nationwide Overview." *International Journal of Radiation: Oncology, Biology, Physics,* vol. 13 (Nov. 1986), pp. 659–663.

Porter, Arthur T., M.D. "Strontium-89 in the Treatment of Bone Metastasis from Prostate Cancer." Paper presented at conference, Prostate Cancer: Detection and Management Controversies in the 1990s, Sutter Cancer Center, Mathews Foundation, Sacramento, Calif., Nov. 6–7, 1992.

———. "The Significance and Implications of Microscopic Residual Local Cancer Following External Beam Radiotherapy." Paper presented at conference, Prostate Cancer: Detection and Management Controversies in the 1990s, Sutter Cancer Center, Mathews Foundation, Sacramento, Calif., Nov. 6–7, 1992.

Porter, Arthur T., M.D., and Jeffrey D. Forman, M.D. "Prostate Brachytherapy—An Overview." *Cancer,* March 1993 (vol. 71), pp. 950–958.

Potosky, Arnold L., et al. "Rise in Prostatic Cancer Incidence Associated with Increased Use of Transurethral Resection." *Journal of the Na-*

tional Cancer Institute (Reports section), vol. 82, no. 20 (Oct. 17, 1990), pp. 1624–1628.

Prostate Cancer: Pathology, Detection, and Diagnosis. American Cancer Society, Professional Education Publication, 1990. Reprinted from *Ca—A Cancer Journal for Clinicians,* vol. 39 (1989), pp. 325–393.

Radiation Therapy and You: A Guide to Self-Help during Treatment. U.S. Public Health Service, National Institutes of Health, National Cancer Institute, Bethesda, Md. NIH, NCI Publication No. 88-2227. Revised Jan. 1985, reprinted Nov. 1987.

Radiology and Imaging Letter. "Improved MR Imaging: Multiple Coils." Vol. 11, no. 9 (May 15, 1991), pp. 65–66.

———. "Prostate Cancer Screening: Digital Exam, Ultrasound, and Antigen Assay." Vol. 11, no. 14 (Aug. 1, 1991), pp. 106–107.

Resnick, Martin I., M.D. "Prostate Cancer and Radiation Therapy" (editorial). *Contemporary Urology,* Feb. 1993, p. 8.

Richie, Jerome P., M.D., and Charles B. Brendler, M.D. (symposium co-directors). *Carcinoma of the Prostate.* Report of symposium, Nov. 15–17, 1991, Orlando, Fla. American Urological Association Office of Education, 1991.

Richie, Jerome P., M.D., et al. (nine-institution study). "Effect of Patient Age on Early Detection of Prostate Cancer with Serum Prostate-Specific Antigen and Digital Rectal Examination." *Urology,* vol. 42, no. 4 (Oct. 1993), pp. 365–374.

Rous, Stephen N., M.D. *The Prostate Book: Sound Advice on Symptoms and Treatment.* Mt. Vernon, N.Y.: Consumers Union, Oct. 1989; update, Norton, 1992.

Scardino, Peter T., M.D., et al. "Early Diagnosis of Prostate Cancer Vital to Cure the Disease." *A.U.A. Today,* vol. 4, no. 9 (Sept. 1991).

Scher, Howard, M.D. "Prostatic Cancer: Where Do We Go from Here?" *Current Science* 1991; reprinted in *Current Opinion in Oncology,* vol. 3 (1991), pp. 568–574.

Schover, Leslie R., Ph.D. "Sexual Rehabilitation after Treatment for Prostate Cancer." *Cancer,* vol. 71, supplement (1993), pp. 1024–1030.

Schover, Leslie R., Ph.D.; Drogo K. Montague, M.D.; and Wendy S. Schain, Ed.D. "Supportive Care and the Quality of Life of the Cancer Patient: Sexual Problems." In *Cancer: Principles and Practice of Oncology,* 3d ed., ed. V. T. DeVita, S. Hellman, and S. A. Rosenberg, pp. 2206–2225. Philadelphia: Lippincott, 1989.

Schwartz, Charles. "Implants for Treatment of Prostate Cancer." *Us Too* (Prostate Cancer Support Group newsletter), vol. 1, no. 4 (Aug./Sept. 1993), pp. 1, 3.

Servadio, Ciro, M.D., et al. "Fifteen Years Experience of Combined Hormone/Chemotherapy in Metastatic Prostate Cancer." *Urology*, vol. 39, no. 3 (Mar. 1992), pp. 274–276.

Severson, Richard K., Ph.D. "Have Transurethral Resections Contributed to the Increasing Incidence of Prostate Cancer?" (editorial). *Journal of the National Cancer Institute*, vol. 82, no. 20 (Oct. 17, 1990), pp. 1597–1598.

Smith, Joseph A., M.D. "Local Recurrence after Radical Prostatectomy." *Us Too* (Prostate Cancer Support Group newsletter), vol. 1, no. 4 (Aug./Sept. 1993), p. 2.

————, guest editor. *The Urologic Clinics of North America*, vol. 17, no. 4 (Nov. 1990), *Early Detection and Treatment of Localized Carcinoma of the Prostate.*

Soloway, Mark S., M.D.; Joseph A. Smith, Jr., M.D.; et al. "Zoladex versus Orchiectomy in Treatment of Advanced Prostate Cancer: A Randomized Trial." *Urology*, vol. 38, no. 1 (Jan. 1991), pp. 46–51.

Stamey, Thomas A., M.D. "Early Detection of Prostate Cancer: A Guide to Screening." *A.U.A. Today*, vol. 4, no. 9 (Sept. 1991), pp. 4, 11.

Stamey, Thomas A., M.D., et al. "Prostate Specific Antigen as a Serum Marker for Adenocarcinoma of the Prostate." *New England Journal of Medicine*, vol. 317, no. 15 (Oct. 8, 1987), pp. 909–916.

Stein, Avi, M.D., et al. "Adjuvant Radiotherapy in Patients Post-Radical Prostatectomy with Tumor Extending through Capsule or Positive Seminal Vesicles." *Urology*, vol. 39, no. 1 (Jan. 1992), pp. 59–62.

Summers, Jack L., M.D. "Maintaining Sexual Function after Radical Prostatectomy." *A.U.A. Today*, vol. 4, no. 9 (Sept. 1991), p. 9.

Torti, Frank M., M.D., guest ed.; Alan J. Wein, M.D., and Bruce Malkowicz, series eds. *Controversies in the Management of Prostate Cancer*, part 5: *Alternatives in Treatment.* Philadelphia: CoMed Communications, General Medical Publications, 1991.

University of California at Berkeley Wellness Letter. "PSA Test: How Well Does It Detect Prostate Cancer?" vol. 9, no. 11 (Aug. 1993), pp. 1–2.

Walsh, P. C., M.D. "Radical Retropubic Prostatectomy." In *Campbell's Urology*, 5th ed., pp. 2654–2775. Philadelphia: W. B. Saunders, 1986.

————. "Radical Retropubic Prostatectomy with Reduced Morbidity: An Anatomical Approach." *NCI Monographs*, no. 7 (1988). NIH Publication no. 88-3005.

Walsh, P. C., M.D., and Pieter J. Donker, M.D. "Impotence Following Radical Prostatectomy—Insight into Etiology and Prevention." *Journal of Urology*, vol. 128 (Sept. 1982), pp. 492–497.

Walsh, P. C., M.D.; Hebert Lepor, M.D.; and J. C. Eggleton, M.D. "Radical Prostatectomy with Preservation of Sexual Function: Anatomical and Pathological Considerations." In *The Prostate*, vol. 4, pp. 473–483. (Reprints: Dr. Patrick Walsh, Brady Urological Institute, Johns Hopkins Hospital, Baltimore, MD 21205.)

Walsh, P. C., M.D., and J. L. Mostwin, M.D. "Radical Prostatectomy and Cystoprostatectomy with Preservation of Potency: Results Using a New Nerve-Sparing Technique." *British Journal of Urology*, vol. 56 (1984), pp. 694–697.

Wang, M. C., et al. "Purification of a Human Prostate Specific Antigen." *Investigative Urology*, vol. 17, no. 2 (Sept. 1979), pp. 159–163.

Warner, John A., M.D., F.R.C.S.(C), and W. D. W. Heston, Ph.D. "Future Developments of Nonhormonal Systemic Therapy for Prostatic Carcinoma." *Urologic Clinics of North America*, vol. 18, no. 1 (Feb. 1991), pp. 25–33.

Weems, W. Lamar, M.D. Interview with Dr. Joseph E. Oesterling, special section on prostate cancer, *Urology Times*, vol. 21, no. 9 (Sept. 1993).

Werthman, Philip, M.D., et al. "Carcinoma of Prostate in Men Aged Fifty and Under: Therapeutic Options." *Urology*, vol. 39, no. 1 (Jan. 1992), pp. 48–51.

What You Need to Know about Prostate Cancer. National Institutes of Health, National Cancer Institute, NIH Publication No. 90-1576. April, 1990.

White, Ralph deVere, M.D., et al. "Urinary Prostate Specific Antigen Levels: Role in Monitoring the Response of Prostate Cancer to Therapy." *Journal of Urology*, vol. 147 (Mar. 1992), pp. 947–951.

Whitmore, Willet F., Jr., M.D. "Conservative Approaches to the Management of Localized Prostate Cancer." Address delivered at American Cancer Society National Conference on Prostate Cancer, Feb. 1992.

———. "Management of Clinically Localized Prostate Cancer: An Unresolved Problem" (editorial). *Journal of the American Medical Association*, vol. 269, no. 20 (May 26, 1993), pp. 2676–2677.

Whitmore, Willet F., Jr., M.D., et al. "Expectant Management of Localized Prostate Cancer." *Cancer*, vol. 67, no. 4 (Feb. 15, 1991), pp. 1091–1096.

Zagars, Gunar K., M.D., and Andrew C. von Eschenbach, M.D. "Management of Clinically Localized Adenocarcinoma of the Prostate: Radiotherapy vs. Surgery." *Cancer Bulletin*, vol. 41, no. 2 (1989), pp. 94–97.

Zagars, Gunar K., M.D.; Andrew C. von Eschenbach, M.D.; D. E. Johnson; and M. J. Oswald. "Stage C Localized Adenocarcinoma: An

Analysis of 551 Patients Treated with External Beam Radiation." *Cancer,* vol. 60 (1987), pp. 1489–1499.

Zietman, A. L., M.D.; J. J. Coen, B.A.; W. U. Shipley, M.D.; and A. F. Althausen, M.D. "Adjuvant Irradiation after Radical Prostatectomy for Adenocarcinoma of the Prostate: Analysis of Freedom from PSA Failure." *Urology,* vol. 42, no. 3 (Sept. 1993), pp. 292–299.

Zincke, Horst, M.D. "Radical Prostatectomy and Exenteractive Procedures for Local Failure after Radiotherapy with Curative Intent: Comparison of Outcomes." *Journal of Urology,* vol. 147 (Mar. 1992), pp. 894–899.

Index